THE TOXICOLOGY OF RADIOACTIVE SUBSTANCES

VOLUME 4

Thorium-232 and Uranium-238

THE TOXICOLOGY OF RADIOACTIVE SUBSTANCES

VOLUME 4

Thorium-232 and Uranium-238

Edited by

A. A. LETAVET

and

E. B. KURLYANDSKAYA

Translated by

A. CROZY

Translation edited by

G. W. DOLPHIN

UNITED KINGDOM ATOMIC ENERGY AUTHORITY
Authority Health and Safety Branch
Radiological Protection Division, Harwell

1966

PERGAMON PRESS

OXFORD · LONDON · EDINBURGH · NEW YORK
TORONTO · SYDNEY · PARIS · BRAUNSCHWEIG

Pergamon Press Ltd., Headington Hill Hall, Oxford
4 & 5 Fitzroy Square, London W.1
Pergamon Press (Scotland) Ltd., 2 & 3 Teviot Place, Edinburgh 1
Pergamon Press Inc., Maxwell House, Fairview Park, Elmsford, New York 10523
Pergamon of Canada Ltd., 207 Queen's Quay West, Toronto 1
Pergamon Press (Aust.) Pty. Ltd., 19a Boundary Street, Rushcutters Bay, N.S.W. 2011, Australia
Pergamon Press S.A.R.L., 24 rue des Écoles, Paris 5e
Vieweg & Sohn GmbH, Burgplatz 1, Braunschweig

First English edition 1970

Library of Congress Catalog Card No. 61-9783

This is a translation of the original Russian published in 1964 by Medgiz, Moscow

Printed in Hungary

08 013413 0

CONTENTS

CERTAIN ASPECTS OF THE TOXICOLOGY OF INSOLUBLE COMPOUNDS OF THORIUM-232 AND URANIUM-238

E. B. KURLYANDSKAYA

STUDY of the toxicity of the natural radioactive substances thorium-232 and uranium-238 is an important practical and theoretical task. Theoretical interest in the problems of the toxicology of thorium and uranium is determined by the dual nature of the biological effects of these elements on entry into the body. The point is that early biological effects produced by these substances are the result of their genuine chemical toxicity, whereas the late ones, as a rule, depend on the radioactivity of the compounds of thorium and uranium.

The literature contains quite a considerable volume of information characterizing the toxic properties of soluble and insoluble compounds of these elements. Thus, McClinton *et al.* (1948) consider that the LD_{50} of soluble thorium nitrate on intraperitoneal injection into rats is 68 mg/kg (calculated for thorium) and its tolerated dose 48·6 mg/kg. According to Watanabe (1957) the mean lethal dose of thorium chloride injected intravenously into mice is 44·3 mg/kg and the tolerated dose 5 mg/kg.

The insoluble salts of thorium-232 are distinguished by low toxicity as indicated by the considerable clinical material accumulated as a result of use of colloidal thorium dioxide (Thorotrast) for radiodiagnosis. At late stages after administration, the radiotoxic properties of Thorotrast became manifest, producing a rather high incidence of neoplasma in the parenchymatous organs rich in reticulo-endothelial elements. The same also applies to uranium compounds. The high toxicity of the nitrates, chlorides and other soluble compounds of uranium is known and was already described in 1889 (Woroschilsky, 1889). According to Haven and Hodge (1949) the intraperitoneal rat LD_{50} for uranium nitrate is 2·37 mg/kg (1·12 mg/kg calculated for uranium) and the equivalent for rabbits 2 mg/kg (0·95 mg/kg for uranium). These findings indicate the high toxicity of soluble compounds of uranium. Its insoluble compounds (UO_2, U_3O_8) are considerably less toxic, according to Dygert *et al.* (1949). Pathological lesions are also seen at late times after administration of these compounds, which may be connected with the alpha-activity of uranium.

Despite the considerable importance of thorium and uranium as will be discussed in detail in the relevant papers in the present volume and despite the attention which in the last few years has been paid to the toxicology of these elements, we still lack sufficiently convincing data on the behaviour of their various compounds, their biological effects and also the late sequelae of their administration. This is especially the case for the insoluble compounds.

The present collection presents material from experimental investigations carried out in the radiotoxicology laboratory of the Institute of Labour Hygiene and Occupational Diseases, U.S.S.R. Academy of Medical Sciences, and devoted to certain aspects of the toxicology of insoluble compounds of these elements, namely, thorium dioxide ($^{232}ThO_2$) and uranous-uranic oxide ($^{238}U_3O_8$).

To establish the toxicity of thorium dioxide, Yan Syao-Shan compared it with the soluble compounds thorium nitrate and chloride. It was found that the most toxic is thorium nitrate, the $LD_{50/30}$ of which on intraperitoneal injection in mice is 370·8 mg/kg (calculated for thorium). According to Traikovich, intracardiac administration of 1 mg/kg thorium nitrate causes instant death of rats as a result of embolism by coagulated proteins. The least toxicity is shown by thorium dioxide, the minimum lethal dose of which is about 2000 mg/kg.

The comparative data on the behaviour of soluble and insoluble compounds of thorium for different routes of administration are of definite interest. Thus, the investigations carried out by Traikovich show that on intracardiac administration of thorium citrate to rats the greatest amount of thorium is found in organs rich in reticulo-endothelial elements—the liver and spleen (17 and 3 per cent of the thorium administered). For the intraperitoneal, intramuscular and oral routes, 53–75 per cent of the amount found in the body was detected in the bones (about 2 per cent of that administered). A large amount of thorium was at the site of administration apparently connected with the formation of poorly soluble complexes which are fixed there for a long time.

Different behaviour is shown by thorium dioxide. As shown by the investigations of Yan Syao-Shan, thorium dioxide is retained for a long time in the lungs on intratracheal and in the abdominal cavity on intraperitoneal administration. Thus, in the early stages after administration of thorium dioxide from 68 to 73 per cent is found in the lungs and after 21 months up to 30 per cent of that administered. Only in the first few days after intratracheal administration was thorium dioxide found in the trachea, lymph nodes, gastro-intestinal tract, liver, bones and kidneys.

Up to 75 per cent of the thorium dioxide administered was found in the abdominal cavity 15 months after intraperitoneal injection. Some was found in the mesenterial lymph nodes and also about 0·33–0·51 per cent of the amount administered was in the bones.

These findings show that a certain part of the thorium dioxide administered is dissolved in body fluids. Possible evidence of this is the presence of thorium in the bones and also its excretion in the urine. Some of the thorium dioxide may be removed by the phagocytes and is held in the reticulo-endothelial tissue. But the fraction of thorium dioxide retained by the organs and the tissues is negligible as compared with the amount fixed at the site of administration. In line with the low true toxicity of thorium dioxide the changes in the rat body at early times (during 10–12 months) after intratracheal and intraperitoneal administration are slight and differ little from those observed in control animals. In rats given 2 and 20 mg/kg thorium dioxide intratracheally (first and second groups) the counts of the peripheral blood cells were not outside normal limits for a long period. Only in individual animals of these groups was it possible, 10–14 months after intratracheal administration, to note transient anaemia accompanied by considerable reticulocytosis. Marked change in erythropoiesis was noted only in rats given high doses of thorium dioxide (300–400 mg/kg). In the animals of these groups (third and fourth), starting from 6 weeks and especially 3 and 6 months after administration of ThO_2, a considerable number of cases of marked reticulopenia were observed with a reticulocyte count at about 0·9 per cent and lower. Thus, changes in erythropoiesis are related to dose.

Some depression of leucopoiesis was noted in rats of the third group in the 7th and 9th months and in animals of the fourth group in the 4th month. Cytological changes in the leucocytes were seen before numerical ones. These changes (fragmentation of the nuclei of the neutrophils, hypersegmentation and chromatinolysis) were of the degenerative-destructive character, but also were possibly associated with disturbances in the processes of maturation of the neutrophils.

The number of lymphocytes fell considerably after 7–8 months in rats given 200 mg/kg thorium dioxide and in rats of the fourth group (300 mg/kg), 3 months after administration. Together with the numerical, morphological changes were seen in vacuolization of the protoplasm, and sometimes also of the nuclei of the lymphocytes. At later stages, binucleated lymphocytes appeared as a result of amitotic cell division. Changes in thrombocytopoiesis reflected in thrombocytosis appeared only in rats which had received 200 mg/kg and more thorium dioxide.

Thus, at late stages after intratracheal administration of thorium dioxide changes in erythropoiesis and leucopoiesis appeared similar to those observed as a result of oral administration of radioactive isotopes (Beloborodova and Baranova, 1957; Beloborodova, 1960; Beloborodova, Ponomareva and Red'kina, 1962; Sagaidak *et al.*, 1962; and others). The character of these changes and the late times of their appearance allow us to relate them to the radioactivity of thorium dioxide.

A characteristic late effect of the biological action of thorium dioxide according to Yan Syao-Shan is seen in the fall in arterial pressure in rats given thorium dioxide via the intratracheal and intraperitonal routes. No distinct relation was established between the fall in arterial pressure and the dose of thorium given. The difference was only in the times of appearance of hypotension. Thus, in the rats which received from 2 to 200 mg/kg thorium dioxide it appeared in the period from 11 to 12 months and for higher doses (300, 400 and 1000 mg/kg) 6–7 months after administration.

It should be noted that after intraperitoneal injection of high doses of thorium dioxide the fall in blood pressure set in later than for intratracheal administration. Possibly this is connected with the huge receptor surface of the lungs, irritation of which causes considerable disturbances in the regulation of blood circulation. Such a reaction of the vascular system appearing at late stages after administration of thorium dioxide may also be related to the radiation effect of thorium since from the numerous experimental and clinical findings it is known that ionizing radiations produce hypotension.

The function of the central nervous system was quite stable inasmuch as it can be judged from the threshold of stimulation of the neuromuscular apparatus of a hind paw of the rat. During 18 months' observation no significant changes were observed which could be linked with the action of thorium dioxide. It is possible that use of more refined methods might reveal changes in the functional state of the central nervous system. Nevertheless, these findings suggest absence of organic lesions of the central nervous system in the conditions of our experiment as indicated by the results of pathomorphological investigation.

Of great interest are the results of the morphological investigations carried out by Gaidova and Yan Syao-Shan. It was found that a single administration of thorium dioxide produces histological lesions in the lungs and the parenchymatous organs, directly related to the dose of substance administered. The most serious lesions were observed in the lungs. They appeared on intratracheal injection of thorium dioxide and were of a uniform nature. They were manifest in the development of suppurative processes in the bronchi, with sclerotic changes in the peribronchial tissue, development of pneumonia, abscesses and adenomatous proliferations. At late stages, after 13–21 months, 13·6 per cent of the test rats had developed tumours which proved to be sarcomas or squamous cell cancer of the lungs. The minimum dose at which the first tumours were seen was 2 mg/kg body weight which corresponds to an activity of $19{\cdot}2 \times 10^{-5}$ μCi per kg body weight.

Histoautography revealed tracks of the path of alpha-particles and stellate figures in the lung tissues of these rats 13–18 months after administration of thorium dioxide.

All this suggests that thorium dioxide possesses low true toxicity so that even for high doses (intratracheal and intraperitoneal) no marked changes are found in the early stages after administration. The late biological effects such as changes in the peripheral blood, reduction in blood pressure and appearance of neoplasms corresponds to those produced by internal and external irradiation with different ionizing radiation sources.

All this and also the fact that the neoplasms appear on intratracheal administration of low doses exceeding only ten times the maximum permissible ones for single administration of thorium dioxide places it in the category of one of the most toxic radioactive substances, which is also confirmed by the considerable experience with the clinical diagnostic use of colloidal thorium dioxide (Thorotrast).

In the present collection we have considered it pertinent to include a description of the technique of determination of thorium in biological media devised by Pavlovskaya and Cherkashina, since the high sensitivity of this technique made it possible to obtain reliable quantitative data on the thorium contents of various biological media. This technique may be useful for those working with thorium.

The review also contains laboratory studies on the acute and chronic effects of the very poorly soluble uranium compound U_3O_8. These investigations were carried out in 1947–50 and prompted work in the radiotoxicology laboratory on the comparative effects of soluble and insoluble compounds of radioactive substances among which a place must be assigned to uranium.

The published findings on toxicity of uranous-uranic oxide (U_3O_8) are few. The work of Haven and Hodge (1949) and Dygert *et al.* (1951) by no means exhausted all the problems of the toxicology of this compound and the observation period was merely a month.

The investigations of Rubanovskaya showed that negligible amounts of U_3O_8 are absorbed in the gastro-intestinal tract of the order of hundredths and thousandths of a per cent of the amount given judged by the urinary excretion of uranium and its content in the kidneys. Consequently, dogs given by mouth a total dose of 17–100 g of this compound over a long time remained practically healthy and U_3O_8 was almost completely removed via the gastro-intestinal tract. Determinable amounts of uranium were found only in the kidneys and thyroid.

As shown by the investigations of Beloborodova in these dogs no changes in the red blood cells were found. The white cells tended to show neutrophilesis. The absolute numbers of lymphocytes and monocytes rose. The morphological investigations of Tolgskaya revealed some hyperplasia of the reticulo-endothelial cells of the spleen and lymph nodes. In the kidneys a minor degenerative process was observed and local circulation disturbances in the walls of the intestines.

The results suggest that U_3O_8 has low but marked toxicity which despite the insignificant absorption of this compound in the gastro-intestinal tract is manifest at different times of treatment. Unfortunately, our investigations were confined to observations for one year which prevented us from following up these animals at late stages when they might have shown a radiation effect from the U_3O_8 given.

The findings on intratracheal injection of U_3O_8 to rabbits and dogs are of interest. In these conditions of administration uranium was found for a long time in the lungs. The investigations of Rubanovskaya showed that over a long period the lungs are cleared of particles of U_3O_8. For example, 4–9 days after intratracheal administration from 53–79 per cent of the amount of U_3O_8 administered was found in the lungs of rabbits. Similar amounts of thorium dioxide were found in rats at the same times after intratracheal administration. After 2·5 months from 15–53 per cent U_3O_8 was detected in the rabbits and after 5·5 to 10 months from 5·5 to 35·6 per cent of the amount given (about 10–50 per cent of the amount found in the lungs in the first days).

Thus, during 10 months' observation uranium was removed from the lungs. The latter was found only in small amounts in the urine and faeces. It is possible that such vigorous excretion of uranium from the lungs is connected with the fact that, as shown by the investigations of Tolgskaya, large accumulations of uranium granules are freely situated in the lumens of the alveoli and in the interalveolar septa. The reaction of the surrounding connective tissue is weakly marked and no nodular formations of a connective tissue character appear as found, for example, for quartz dust. The absence of a marked fibrous reaction is possibly connected with the radioactivity of uranium. The appearance in the pulmonary tissue of foreign body cells around the accumulations of uranium is also characteristic. The catarrhal-desquamative inflammatory process in the lungs is highly marked.

Intratracheal administration of considerable amounts of U_3O_8 (up to 1 g) in dogs causes acute poisoning similar to that described by Woroschilsky in 1889 for the soluble uranium salts. These animals 10–12 days after administration of U_3O_8 develop severe lesions, chiefly of the kidneys, which we do not observe on oral administration even of high amounts (up to

100 g). These findings show that in relation to the chemical toxicity, intratracheal injection of insoluble uranium compounds presents considerable hazards.

Tolgskaya presents a detailed morphological description of acute and chronic involvement in rabbits and dogs on oral and intratracheal administration of U_3O_8. The main changes were found by her in the lungs, kidneys, the subcortical nodes of the thalamo-hypothalamic region and in the medulla oblongata with insignificant changes in the cerebral cortex and other organs.

The investigations of Kurlyandskaya were concerned with the permeability of the placenta for U_3O_8, the possibility of its excretion by the mammary glands and also the influence of this compound on intra-uterine foetal development and in the early post-natal period. These investigations showed that following oral and intratracheal administration of the virtually insoluble uranium compound to the pregnant animal, uranium is found in the placenta and foetal tissues. It is also found in the milk of lactating animals and in the tissues and urine of puppies and rabbits fed with the milk of females burdened with uranium.

Prolonged observation of the state and development of animals exposed to the chronic action of U_3O_8 and their progeny established that it exerts a certain effect on the reproductive ability of the females and on the uterine and early post-natal development of rabbits and dogs. The findings obtained concur with those described by Maynard and Hodge (1949) who found a reduction in the litter size for rats exposed to the chronic action of uranium nitrate.

Our laboratory findings on the toxicology of U_3O_8 do not diverge from those of Dygert *et al.* (1951) who showed that inhalation of U_3O_8 in considerable concentrations (20 mg/m^3) may cause heavy damage to the kidneys and even death.

On the basis of the results we may judge chiefly the chemical toxicity of U_3O_8 since the observation times, as stated above, were not long enough to detect radiation damage in rabbits and dogs. This is due to the low specific activity of uranium and the consequent need for a longer time for the onset of the late sequelae as occurs in rats following the intratracheal administration of thorium dioxide.

The short review given in the present paper far from exhausts all the aspects of the toxicology of the oxide of thorium-232 and uranous-uranic 238-uranium, which are detailed in the papers in the present collection. Its purpose was to give some generalizations and sharpen awareness of certain patterns important for the understanding of the toxicology of these substances.

References

BELOBORODOVA N. L. and BARANOVA YE. F., Radiotoxic Effect of ^{89}Strontium under the Conditions of a Continuous Experiment (Radiotoksicheskoye deistviye radioaktivnogo strontsiya v usloviyakh khronicheskogo eksperimenta). In: *Toxicology of Radioactive Substances* (*Materialy po toksikologii radioaktivnykh veshchesty*), Vol. 1, p. 151. Moscow (1957).

BELOBORODOVA N. L. and BARANOVA YE. F., Changes in the Peripheral Blood and Certain Other Factors on Continuous Administration of Radioactive Caesium (Izmeneniya perifericheskoi krovi i nekotorykh drugikh pokazatelei pri khronicheskom vozdeistvii radioaktivnogo tseziya). *Ibid.*, p. 162.

BELOBORODOVA N. L. and BARANOVA YE. F., Effect on Haemopoiesis of Prolonged Oral Administration of Radioactive Ruthenium (Vliyaniye na krovotvoreniye dlitel'nogo vvedeniya cherez rot radioaktivnogo ruteniya). *Ibid.*, p. 166.

BELOBORODOVA N. L. and BARANOVA YE. F., Investigation of the Functional State of the Haemopoietic System in Rabbits subjected to Continuous Administration of Radioactive Caesium, Strontium and Ruthenium (Issledovaniye funktsional'nogo sostoyaniya krovotvornoi sistemy u krolikov, podvergavshikhaya khronicheskomu vozdeistviyu radioaktivnogo tseziya, stronttsiya i ruteniya). *Ibid.*, p. 171.

BELOBORODOVA N. L., Changes in Haemopoiesis during Prolonged Internal Administration of ^{60}Co (Izmeneniye protsessov krovotvoreniya pri dlitel'nom vvedenii vnutr' Co^{60}). In: *Toxicology of Radioactive Substances*, Vol. 2, p. 39. Moscow (1960).

BELOBORODOVA N. L., PONOMAREVA V. L. and RED'KINA E. K., The Effect of Prolonged ^{59}Fe Administration on Haemopoiesis (Krovotvoreniye pri khronicheskom deistvii Fe^{59}). In: *Toxicology of Radioactive Substances*, Vol. 3, p. 48. Moscow (1962).

DYGERT H. P., LABELLE C. W., LASKIN S., POZZANI U. C., ROBERTS E., ROTHERMEL J. J., ROTHSTEIN A., SPIEGL C. J., SPRAGUE G. F. and STOCKINGER H. E., Toxicity following Inhalation (Toksichnost' uranovykh soyedinenii pri ingalyassionnom vvedenii). In: *The Pharmacology and Toxicology of Uranium Compounds*, Vol. 1, p. 423. Foreign Literature Publishing House, Moscow (1951).

HAVEN F. and HODGE H. C., Toxicity following Parenteral Administration of Certain Soluble Uranium Salts. In: *Pharmacology and Toxicology of Uranium Compounds*, Vol. 1, p. 281. McGraw-Hill, New York (1949).

MAYNARD E. A. and HODGE H. C., Studies of Toxicity of Various Uranium Compounds when fed to Experimental Animals. In: *Pharmacology and Toxicology of Uranium Compounds*, Vol. 1, p. 309. McGraw-Hill, New York (1949).

McCLINTON L. T. and SCHUBERT J., The Toxicity of Some Zirconium and Thorium Salts in Rats. *J. Pharm. Exp. Ther.* **94**, 1 (1948).

PONOMAREVA V. L., Changes in Erythropoiesis during Prolonged Administration of ^{59}Fe (K voprosu ob izmeneniyakh eritropoeza pri dlitel'nom vozdeistvii Fe^{59}). In: *Toxicology of Radioactive Substances*, Vol. 3, p. 56. Moscow (1962).

POZZANI J., Vysokokachestvennaya ruda (High-grade Ore). In: *The Pharmacology and Toxicology of Uranium Compounds*, Vol. 2, p. 115. Foreign Literature Publishing House, Moscow (1951).

SAGAIDAK N. D., Peripheral Blood Changes in White Rats following Intratracheal Injection of Various ^{59}Fe Compounds (Izmeneniya perifericheskoi krovi pri intratrakheal'nom vvedenii belykh krysam razlichnykh soyedinenii Fe^{59}). In: *Toxicology of Radioactive Substances*, Vol. 3, p. 86. Moscow (1962).

WATANABE S., Pharmacological and Toxicological Studies on Thorium, a Rare Earth Metal. *J. Tokyo Med. College* **15**, No. 2, 121–439 (1957).

WOROSCHILSKY L., Wirkung des Urans. Diss., Dorpat (1889).

COMPARATIVE TOXICITY OF SOLUBLE AND INSOLUBLE COMPOUNDS OF THORIUM-232

YAN SYAO-SHAN

THORIUM, one of the natural radioactive elements, was discovered by Belzelius in 1828 in minerals. After the discovery investigations carried out simultaneously in 1888 by Schmidt and Marie Curie showed that thorium compounds are radioactive and emit rays like those of uranium. In 1900, the emanation of thorium was isolated and in 1905 radiothorium was discovered and in 1907 mesothorium.

With the discovery of nuclear fission and advances in the field of nuclear energetics, namely, the possibility of using thorium for increasing the reserves of fissionable isotopes, interest in the physics and chemistry of thorium sharply increased. This is indicated by the reports presented to the First and Second International Conferences on the Peaceful Uses of Atomic Energy held in Geneva in 1955 and 1958 (Katsin, 1955; Kaplan, 1955; Hayawara, 1958; and others).

In the present paper we give only information on the physical and physico-chemical properties of thorium which in our view is necessary for solving certain problems in radiotoxicology outlined in the present and the following papers in this collection.

Physicochemical Constants for Thorium

Atomic number	90
Atomic weight	232·05
Atomic diameter, Å	3·59
Melting point, °C	1750
Boiling point, °C	3540–4200
Thermal conductivity, cal/cm sec °C	
at 20°C	0·090
at 100°C	0·090
at 600°C	0·106
Work function of electron, eV	3·39
Electrochemical potential of thorium ion (Th^{4+}) in normal conditions	1·90 V

Physicochemical Constants for Thorium Dioxide (according to the *American Refractories Inst. Techn. Bull.* 1956, No. 94)

Density, g/cm^3	9·7
Melting point, °C	3220±16
Boiling point, °C	4400
Thermal conductivity, cal/cm sec °C	
100°C	0·025
500°C	0·014
1200°C	0·0076
Strength at rupture, at room temperature, kg/cm	1000–1260
Dissociation elasticity, atm	
at 2000°C	10^{-27}
at 3000°C	10^{-5}

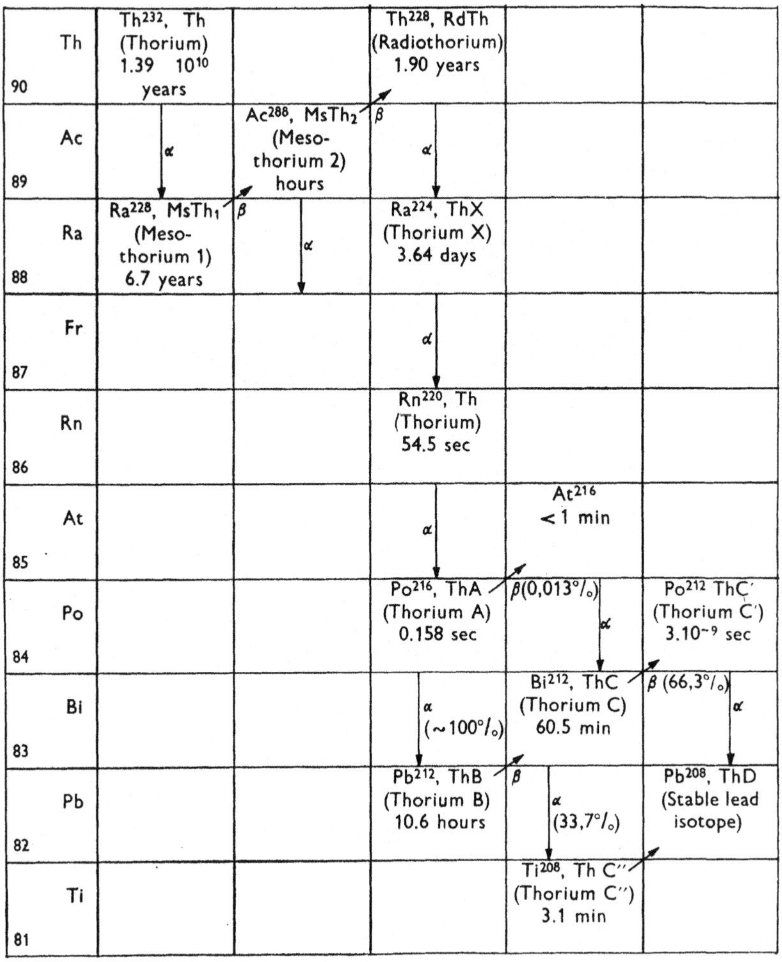

FIG. 1. Scheme of radioactive decay of thorium

Because of the above-listed properties, thorium and thorium dioxide have been widely adopted in various fields of industry. Thus, thorium has a high melting point, does not undergo phase conversions up to 1400°C, possesses a cubic lattice, is stable to irradiation and is a good reactor material (Hayawara, 1958).

In the production of incandescent lamp filaments, addition of thorium dioxide to tungsten stabilizes the structure of the latter and the filaments are given increased vibrational strength. Because of the high yield point and the high stability at raised temperatures of alloys containing thorium, the latter is used in casting compressor parts for reactive engines (*Metal Progress, 71*, No. 2, 1957).

Thus, even this short list of the properties of thorium and the area of its applications shows the exciting possibilities for use of thorium and, consequently, the degree of contact with it in various branches of industry.

Thorium, $^{232}_{90}Th$, is the first element of the radioactive family called after it. The scheme of radioactive decay of thorium is given in Fig. 1.

Natural thorium consists practically of one isotope ^{232}Th with a half-

TABLE 1. *Radioactive Substances of Thorium Family in Radioactive Equilibrium (by weight)*

Name		Half-life in seconds	Mass per g of Th, in grams	Energy in MeV
MsTh	Th 1 Isotope Ra	$4{\cdot}38\times10^{17}$ $2{\cdot}11\times10^{8}$	1·0 $4{\cdot}81\times^{-10}$	$\alpha = 3{\cdot}98$ $\beta = 0{\cdot}053$
MsTh	2 Isotope Ac	$2{\cdot}21\times10^{4}$	$5{\cdot}05\times10^{-14}$	$\beta = 1{\cdot}6$ $\gamma = 0{\cdot}914$
RaTh	Isotope Th	$5{\cdot}99\times10^{7}$	$1{\cdot}37\times10^{-10}$	$\alpha = 5{\cdot}42$ $\gamma = 0{\cdot}085$
ThX	Isotope Ra	$3{\cdot}14\times10^{5}$	$7{\cdot}17\times10^{-13}$	$\alpha = 5{\cdot}861$
Th	Isotope Rn	54·5	$1{\cdot}24+10^{-16}$	$\alpha = 6{\cdot}278$ $\gamma = 0{\cdot}226$
ThA	Isotope Po	0·158	$3{\cdot}61\times10^{-19}$	$\alpha = 6{\cdot}771$
ThB	Isotope Ph	$3{\cdot}82\times10^{4}$	$8{\cdot}72\times10^{-14}$	$\beta = 0{\cdot}36$ $\gamma = 0{\cdot}24$
At	Astatine	3×10^{-4}	$6{\cdot}85\times10^{-22}$	
ThC	Isotope Bi	$3{\cdot}63\times10^{3}$	$8{\cdot}29\times10^{-15}$	$\alpha = 6{\cdot}047$ $\beta = 2{\cdot}26$ $\gamma = 0{\cdot}04$
ThC′	(66·3%) Isotope Po	3×10^{7}	$4{\cdot}51\times10^{-25}$	$\alpha = 8{\cdot}775$
ThC″	(33·7%) Isotope Te	186	$1{\cdot}43\times10^{-16}$	$\beta = 1{\cdot}82$ $\gamma = 2{\cdot}62$

life $T = 1{\cdot}39 \times 10^{10}$ years and daughter decay products in equilibrium with it which account for only a small part of natural thorium.

Data on the amount of radioactive substances of the thorium series present in radioactive equilibrium are presented in Table 1 (Spitsyn, 1955).

One of the most important properties of thorium is that when exposed to neutrons it is converted to the uranium isotope (^{233}U) which serves as a nuclear fuel (Seaborg *et al.*, 1947). This process proceeds according to the following main reaction:

$$^{232}_{90}Th\ (n, \gamma), \longrightarrow {}^{233}_{90}Th\ \beta \longrightarrow {}^{233}_{91}Pu\ \beta \longrightarrow {}^{233}_{92}U$$

Thus, thorium is a potential source for the secondary nuclear fuel $^{233}_{92}U$.

It is known that in the track of alpha particles the greatest density of ionization is produced and therefore, thorium as an alpha emitter with a long half-life, on entering the body may present a serious hazard for persons in contact with it.

The last fifteen years have seen numerous investigations most of which have been concerned with elucidation of the chemical properties of thorium. Previously, thorium was assigned to the second sub-group of the group IV of the periodic system of elements considering it to be an analogue of titanium, zirconium and hafnium. The results of the latest investigations (Seaborg, 1955; Makarov, 1958; Nast *et al.*, 1952; and others) suggest that thorium is the first member of the actinide group. This assumption is confirmed by many facts.

Before 1949 it was considered that thorium showed only a tetravalency (Bietz, 1904; Nilson, 1883) but further investigations showed that in certain conditions thorium may be present also in the bivalent and trivalent states (Anderson, 1949; and others).

Of the numerous complex thorium compounds we most often encounter thorium dioxide (Th_2O) and the nitrate [$Th(NO_3)_4$] and chloride ($ThCl_4$) of thorium. Below are given some of their chemical properties.

Thorium dioxide, depending on the mode of preparation, is crystalline or amorphous. Mild calcination (not above 550–600°C) gives a thorium dioxide which dissolves comparatively readily in acids. Calcined at high temperatures it becomes poorly soluble. Then, its solubility in acids at 25°C is: 2 mg/l. in 1 N H_2SO_4, 0·6 mg/l. in 1 N HNO_3 and 0·5 mg/l. in 1 N HCl (Spitsyn, 1955). Addition of small amounts of fluorine ions speeds the process of solution of ThO_2 in acids. Ryabchikov *et al.* have shown that 0·01–0·05 mole hydrofluoric acid per litre solution rapidly takes into solution thorium dioxide, metallic thorium and other acid-insoluble thorium compounds (Ryabchikov, 1959; Rodden and Wharf, 1956; and others). These findings are important for determining the amount of thorium in biosubstrates, namely, during mineralization and extraction of thorium.

Thorium dioxide virtually does not interact with solutions of caustic alkalis and carbonates of alkaline metals. In 1 litre of water at 25°C less than 0·02 mg thorium dioxide dissolves (Spitsyn, 1917).

Thorium nitrates having several hydrated crystals with a content of up to 12 water molecules are the best soluble of all thorium compounds. Thorium nitrate dissolves well in water but is readily extracted from the aqueous phase with any organic solvents immiscible with the water: alcohols, ketones, simple and complex ethers on addition of nitric acid or another soluble nitrate (Seaborg, 1960).

Thorium chlorides are in the form of white crystals. Crystallization from aqueous solution gives the hydrated crystal $ThCl_4 . 8H_2O$ which on drying loses water turning at 90°C into hydrated thorium tetrachloride and at 120–160°C into the basic chloride $ThOH(Cl_3)H_2O$ and at 250°C into the anhydrous oxychloride $ThOCl_2$ and finally, into ThO_2. The chlorides of thorium dissolve well in water. Products of linkage of thorium chloride with a number of organic substances exist (ethyl and methyl alcohols, acetaldehyde, acetone, etc.).

On interaction of the solutions of the thorium salts with alkalis a gelatinous residue of thorium hydroxide forms. Precipitation of the thorium hydroxide begins in the pH interval from 3·5 to 3·6 irrespective of the concentration of thorium in solution (Seaborg, 1960).

Study of the solubility of thorium and some of its compounds in biosubstrates (Bokova, 1960) showed that in 0·3 per cent hydrochloric acid, close in acidity to gastric juice, metallic thorium dissolves in the following proportion: for 10 mg metallic thorium, 1·1 mg dissolves; for 100 mg, 10–11 mg dissolves; and for 300 mg, 15–16 mg dissolves. The solubility of thorium fluoride in gastric juice is from 16 to 20 per cent and in plasma from 1–2 per cent of the amount taken. Thorium oxide dissolves in these media in smaller amounts than metallic thorium and its fluoride.

The information on thorium-232 presented here far from exhausts the available data on the properties of thorium and its compounds. We consider it necessary to present only material which may prove useful for those working in the field of toxicology of thorium-232. In studying the biological effects of chemical substances which have entered the body it is necessary to have an idea of their toxicity. The latter largely depends on the physicochemical properties of the compounds studied and, in particular, on their solubility in biological fluids.

As stated above, in the industry concerned with extracting and producing thorium the workers mostly have to deal with the oxide (ThO_2), the chloride ($ThCl_4$) and the nitrate [$Th(NO_3)_4$]. The last two compounds of thorium are quite soluble in water. Thorium oxide is practically insoluble. The literature known to us provides very little information on the toxicity of the various thorium compounds. Thus, Tripoli *et al.* (1932) on intravenous injection of Thorotrast in dogs and rabbits and also on intracardiac injection of this compound in guinea-pigs, white mice and rats in doses of 0·8–8·0 g/kg, reported finding in the immediate stages after administration no changes in body weight, the state of the internal organs, appetite or resistance to infection. At later stages animals of the group which received a higher dose of ThO_2 (8·8 g/kg) developed a number of serious lesions. Six of the 75 animals died three days after this dose of Thorotrast. Autopsy revealed foci of necrosis, embolism of the vessels of the spleen and degenerative changes in the kidneys, liver and other organs.

McClinton *et al.* (1948) showed that the mean lethal dose of thorium citrate for rats on intraperitoneal injection is equal (calculated for thorium) to 68 ± 2 mg/kg. The tolerated dose is 48·6 and the absolute lethal dose 157 mg/kg. The solution administered was prepared from thorium nitrate in solution of sodium citrate. The author did not indicate the acidity of solution which has an effect not only on the state of the animal but also on the behaviour of thorium in the body.

Watanabe (1957) pointed out that the mean lethal dose to a mouse of thorium chloride on intravenous injection is 44·3 mg/kg. Intoxication was manifest in inhibited mobility of the animals, increased respiratory rate, tremors, convulsions and paralyses. With the same route of administration the tolerated dose of thorium chloride for rabbits was 5 and the absolute lethal dose 30–35 mg/kg.

On subcutaneous administration of the same solution the tolerated dose was several times higher than the absolute lethal intravenous dose.

Because of the considerable importance of thorium and its compounds in modern industry and also because of the paucity of information on its biological effects we considered it necessary to investigate the comparative toxicity of the most important thorium compounds and establish the main parameters (minimum, absolute and mean lethal doses).

In toxicology to determine the toxicity of chemical substances from the mortality indices the so-called mean lethal dose is used for a definite observation period. For example, the $LD_{50/30}$ is the mean lethal dose for an observation period of 30 days. The LD_{50} has a great advantage in assessing the toxicity of the substance over the absolute lethal dose since it greatly reduces the influence of the individual sensitivity of the animals and the percentage of chance for the findings obtained.

To establish the comparative toxicity we carried out a special investigation. The experiments were carried out on male white mice obtained from the same breeding house and selected by weight (18–20 g). Before administration the mice were kept in the conditions of the animal house for 7 days. In the experiment we used only animals showing no deviations from normal. Administration was via the intraperitoneal route with aqueous solutions of thorium compounds: thorium chloride, nitrate and with suspension of the dioxide. The volume of the solution injected was 0·5 ml. The pH of the solutions of thorium chloride and nitrate were 2–3, of the thorium dioxide suspension 6. In view of the considerable acidity of the solutions injected control animals were injected in parallel by the same route with a solution of 0·01 N HCl, pH 2 or HNO_3 (pH 2–3) or distilled water in a volume of 0·5 ml. A biological check was also run in the experiment. After administration of the thorium compounds the animals were kept under observation in the same way as the controls for 30 days.

For solutions of thorium chloride or nitrate and also after injection of 0·01 N HCl and HNO_3 some of the animals died after 5–10 min. Autopsy at early stages after injection showed engorgement of the internal organs of the abdominal cavity. It is possible that the sharp excitation of the mice which was observed immediately after injection of the thorium compounds was the result of irritation of the abdominal cavity with the acid solution. In the mice injected intraperitoneally with thorium oxide or water no gross lesions were observed.

In the animals which died at later times after injection of solutions of thorium chloride or nitrate, autopsy revealed extensive adhesions of the internal organs of the abdominal cavity. Such phenomena were not seen in the mice given thorium oxide. In these animals macroscopically we found accumulation of thorium oxide in the mesenterium and on the surface of the viscera. No adhesions were noticed in the abdominal cavity of the control mice which received intraperitoneally HCl and HNO_3 at the same pH.

TABLE 2. *Mouse Mortality During 30 Days after Administration of Thorium Nitrate Solution*

Dose in mg/kg		Number of animals	Of them		% mortality
Calculated for $Th(NO_3)_4$	Calculated for Th		Died	Survived	
239	116	10	0	10	0
456	220	20	2	18	10
738	356	20	7	13	35
956	462	20	17	3	85
1200	570	10	10	0	100
1790	866	10	10	0	100
Controls HNO_3 0·5 ml per mouse	0·01 N	10	1	9	10

The details of the mortality of the mice observed for 30 days after injection of the various thorium compounds are presented in Tables 2, 3 and 4.

Table 2 shows that all the animals injected intraperitoneally with thorium nitrate in a dose of about 1200 mg/kg (calculated for thorium 570 mg/kg) died within 30 days of injection. Consequently, this dose is absolutely lethal for white mice. The minimum lethal dose was 456 mg/kg (calculated for thorium 220 mg/kg).

TABLE 3. *Mortality of White Mice During 30 Days after Administration of Thorium Chloride Solution*

Dose in mg/kg		Number of animals	Of them		% mortality
$ThCl_4$	Calculated for Th		Died	Survived	
175	124	13	0	13	0
325	231	10	1	19	10
559	395	10	3	7	30
773	550	10	5	5	50
1265	900	13	11	2	85
1745	1240	13	13	0	100
Controls 0·5 ml HCl per mouse	0·01 N	33	2	31	6

On intraperitoneal injection of the mice with solution of thorium chloride the absolute lethal dose was 1745 mg/kg (for thorium 1240 mg/kg) and the minimum lethal dose 325 mg/kg (231 mg/kg for thorium) (Table 3).

TABLE 4. *Mortality of White Mice During 30 Days after Administration of Thorium Dioxide*

Dose in mg/kg		Number of animals	Of them		% mortality
ThO_2	Calculated for Th		Died	Survived	
226	200	10	0	10	0
565	500	10	0	10	0
1130	1000	10	0	10	0
2250	2000	10	1	9	10
Controls H_2O per mouse,	0·5ml	20	2	18	10
biological controls		30	3	27	10

On administration of thorium oxide suspension the majority of the mice survived even a dose of 2260 mg/kg (2000 mg/kg of thorium) (Table 4).

Table 4 shows that intraperitoneal injection of thorium oxide has very low toxicity as compared with the chloride and nitrate. This is also confirmed by calculation of the mean lethal doses for the thorium compounds (the $LD_{50/30}$) which were estimated from the formula proposed by Pershin:

$$LD_{50/30} = \frac{(a+b)(m-n)}{200}$$

where a and b are doses for adjacent groups,
m and n are mortality in adjacent groups.

According to this calculation the $LD_{50/30}$ for thorium nitrate for white mice is 370·8 mg/kg (calculated for thorium) and for thorium chloride 589·1 mg/kg.

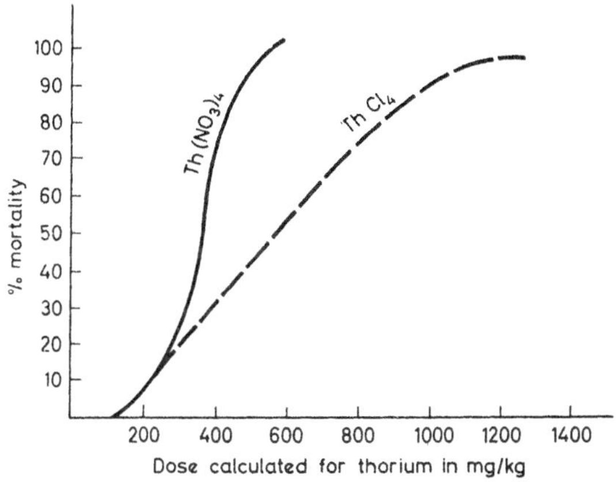

FIG. 2. Mortality curve for white mice given various doses of thorium nitrate and chloride

Thus, in terms of the $LD_{50/30}$ thorium nitrate is most toxic.

The mortality of the mice for different doses of the thorium compounds studied is indicated in Fig. 2 and well illustrates the above remarks.

The findings show that the practically insoluble thorium compound ThO_2 does not cause the death of mice in the first 30 days of intraperitoneal injection, from which it may be concluded that it has low chemical toxicity usually manifest within the period directly following entry of the chemical compound into the body.

Thorium nitrate and chloride display comparatively high toxicity which is manifest early (1–4 days). It may be supposed that the toxicities of these compounds are chiefly connected with their chemical properties since in all the experiments in which the mice were given soluble thorium salts the doses leading to death of the animals were considerably less judging by their thorium content than on administration of the oxide.

Comparing the toxicities of thorium nitrate and chloride it may be seen that the $LD_{50/30}$ for the nitrate is considerably lower than for the chloride. Figure 2 also shows that the range of toxic action of the nitrate is considerably narrower than for thorium chloride which also suggests its higher toxicity.

The difference in the effects of thorium nitrate and chloride may be explained to a certain extent by the higher toxicity of the NO_3 than the Cl ion. This assumption is based on the fact that in control animals receiving 0·01 N HCl the mortality of the white mice was less (6 per cent) than on administration of nitric acid (10 per cent).

Summary

1. Comparative study of the toxic properties of various thorium compounds (nitrate, chloride and oxide) showed that thorium nitrate is most toxic.

2. The difference in the toxicities of the thorium compounds studied is determined by the degree of their solubility and also by the higher toxicity of the NO_3, than the Cl anion. Poorly soluble ThO_2 is least toxic chemically.

References

ANDERSON J. S. *et al.*, The Lower Valency States of Thorium. *J. Chem. Soc.* **2,** 244 (1949).

BELZELIUS *et al.*, *Ann. Phys.* **16,** 385 (1829).

BIETZ W., Quoted by RYABCHIKOV E. K., *Analytical Chemistry of Thorium (Analiticheskaya khimiya toriya)*. Akad. Nauk SSSR, Moscow (1960).

BOKOVA G. B., Study of the Behaviour of Metal Thorium and Some of Its Compounds in Various Media (Izucheniye povedeniya metallicheskogo toriya i nekotorykh ego soyedeninii v razlichnykh sredakh). *Gig. truda i profzabolevanii,* **1,** 49 (1960).

HAYAWARA R. R., Thorium-Uranium Fuel Elements for SRE. Paper No. 785 (U.S.A.) to the Second International Conference on the Peaceful Uses of Atomic Energy, Geneva (1958).

KAPLAN G. E., Metallurgiya toriya (The Metallurgy of Thorium). Paper No. 636 presented to the First International Conference on the Peaceful Uses of Atomic Energy, Geneva (1955).

KATSIN L. I., Posledniye dostizheniya v khimii toriya (The Latest Advances in the Chemistry of Thorium). Paper No. 734 presented to the First International Conference on the Peaceful Uses of Atomic Energy, Geneva (1955).

MAKAROV E. S., *The Crystallochemistry of the Simplest Uranium, Thorium, Plutonium and Neptunium Compounds (Kristallokhimiya prosteishikh soyedinenii urana, toriya, plutoniya i neptuniya)*. Akad. Nauk SSSR, Moscow (1958).

McClinton L. T. and Schubert J., The Toxicity of Some Zirconium and Thorium Salts in Rats. *J. Pharm. Exp. Ther.*, **94,** 1 (1948).

Nast R. and Krakkay T., Quoted by Ryabchikov E. K., *Analytical Chemistry of Thorium*, p. 9. Akad. Nauk USSR (1960).

Nilson L. F., *Ibid.*, p. 10.

Rodden C. J. and Wharf J. C., In: *Analytical Chemistry of Elements Studied on the Manhattan Project.* McGraw-Hill, New York (1950).

Ryabchikov D. P., *Analytical Chemistry of Thorium (Analiticheskaya khimiya toriya).* Akad. Nauk SSSR, Moscow (1960).

Seaborg G. T. and Katz J. J., *The Actinide Elements.* McGraw-Hill, New York (1954).

Seaborg G. T. and Katz J. J., *The Chemistry of Actinide Elements.* Methuen, London (1957).

Seaborg G. T., Gofman J. W. and Stoughton R. W., *Phys. Rev.*, **71,** 378 (1947).

Spitsyn V. I. *et al.*, *Methods of Work with Use of Radioactive Tracers (Metody raboty s primeneniyem radioaktivnykh indikatorov).* Akad. Nauk SSSR, Moscow (1955).

Tripoli C. J. and Haam E. V., Effects of Toxic and Non-toxic Doses in Various Animals. *Proc. Soc. Exp. Biol.* **29**, 1053–1056 (1932).

Watanabe S., Pharmacological and Toxicological Studies on Thorium, a Rare Earth Metal. *J. Tokyo med. College*, **15**, No. 2, 121–139 (1957).

ABSORPTION, DISTRIBUTION AND EXCRETION OF CERTAIN SOLUBLE COMPOUNDS OF NATURAL THORIUM

MIODRAG TRAIKOVICH

THIS paper outlines some information on the distribution and excretion of certain soluble compounds of natural thorium and thorium nitrate in rats after single administration by various routes.

While extensive investigations have been carried out on certain insoluble compounds, especially thorium oxide and Thorotrast, the problem of the soluble compounds of thorium has so far received comparatively little attention and the available evidence is largely of a conflicting character. However, all workers agree that thorium as a chemical element is little toxic especially if it does not directly enter the bloodstream (Yan Syao-Shan, 1962; McClinton and Schubert, 1948; Ackerman *et al.*, 1948). Soluble thorium compounds when directly introduced into the bloodstream accumulate chiefly in the liver, spleen and bone marrow, while following administration by other routes they deposit in bone tissue (Ackerman *et al.*, 1948; Salerno *et al.*, 1951; Scott *et al.*, 1952; Boone *et al.*, 1958; Thomas, 1956). There is lack of agreement on the quantitative data concerning accumulation of thorium in these organs and tissues, the rate of blood clearance, elimination from the body, and so on. In addition, it is difficult to compare data from the various papers since some authors do not describe the experimental technique and do not give the method by which thorium was determined or do not indicate its precision, while others do not describe the method for estimating the amount of thorium administered, and so on.

To elucidate the problems associated with the behaviour of soluble thorium compounds in the body we carried out a number of experiments. These experiments were run on four groups of male white rats with five animals in each group. The mean weight of the rats in the groups was as follows: in the first group 216 g, second 228 g, third 249 g and fourth 323 g. In each group four rats were ear-marked for determination of the content of thorium in the organs and tissues and one for histoautoradiography. We did not run control groups since in the radiotoxicology laboratory of the Institute of Labour Hygiene and Occupational Diseases of the U.S.S.R. Academy of Medical Sciences (Yan Syao-Shan, this volume, p. 34) evidence has been obtained indicating that in normal rats it is impossible to detect even traces of naturally occurring thorium by our method.

All the rats were given thorium nitrate dissolved in saline or in 10 per cent solution of sodium citrate with pH 3·1 and 4·0 respectively. The solutions were administered to the animals by various routes: the first group, intraperitoneally: second, intramuscularly: third, through a stomach tube and the fourth by the intracardiac route. In the first three groups we used a solution of thorium nitrate in saline, in the fourth, in sodium citrate. The first, second and fourth groups received 25 mg of thorium and the third group 50 mg of thorium per rat. It should be noted that intracardiac injection of thorium nitrate led to rapid death of nearly all the animals. Of five rats in this group only one survived.

After administration each rat was placed in a metabolic cage for collection of faeces and urine. At 72 hr the animals were killed by decapitation. In each group we determined on four rats the content of thorium in the organs and tissues; in the blood, liver, spleen, kidneys and in the compact part of the femoral bones (diaphysis) and in the muscles and also in the urine and faeces collected over the 72 hr. To determine the still unabsorbed thorium from the site of administration we took: for intramuscular injection the intact hind limb; for intraperitoneal, the whole of the abdominal part of the trunk together with contents (apart from the liver, spleen and kidneys in which the amounts of thorium were determined separately) and for the oral route, all the gastro-intestinal tract plus contents.

To determine thorium we used the photocolorimetric method of Kuznetsov and Savvin (1961) modified for biological material by Pavlovskaya and Cherkashina (the technique and the advantages of this method are described in a separate paper in this volume). Histoautoradiography was carried out by the method of mounting on A-2 photographic plates proposed by Erleksova (1960).

Determination of thorium in the liver and spleen after intraperitoneal injection presented special difficulties since with this mode of injection deposition of thorium on the surface of these organs cannot be excluded. According to published findings thorium injected intraperitoneally is deposited in the peritoneal and subperitoneal tissues (Scott *et al.*, 1952). Although these findings were obtained in experiments with thorium sulphate it may be supposed that the nitrate behaves similarly. Because of this it was necessary in work with these organs to take a number of measures to prevent passage of thorium from the surface deep into the tissue. Therefore, in removing the organs from the abdominal cavity we tried not to damage their surface. They were washed with running distilled water and then with 0·5 per cent HCl solution. The surface of these organs was rubbed with the same solution and dried. The liver was frozen and cut into pieces 2 mm thick. The external parts of these slices (1 mm thick) were cut off and discarded and only the internal areas were used to determine the thorium content. On treatment of the spleen we confined ourselves to washing with 0·5 per cent HCl and used the spleen as a whole.

The distribution of thorium in the rat organs and tissues for different routes of administration is shown in Table 1, where it will be seen that the content of thorium per gram of tissue for the first three modes of administration was roughly the same. An appreciable difference is shown by the findings only for the liver and spleen of the rats of the first group where a high concentration of thorium was found. It is possible that despite precautionary measures taken, as indicated above, these organs were contaminated, especially if we take into account their large surface in direct

TABLE 1. *Distribution of Thorium in Rat Organs and Tissues for Different Routes of Administration (Mean for 4 Rats)*

Group	Route	Thorium administered	Chemical compound
First	Intraperitoneally	25 mg	Thorium nitrate
Second	Intramuscularly	25 mg	Thorium nitrate
Third	Orally	25 mg[1]	Thorium nitrate
Fourth	Intracardiac	25 mg 10 mg	Thorium nitrate Thorium citrate

Amount of thorium γ per g tissue $\pm\sigma$						
Group	Liver	Spleen	Kidneys	Blood	Muscle	Bone
First	35·45$\mp$ 10·11	21·45$\pm$ 8·30	0·62$\pm$ 0·01	0·99$\pm$ 0·24	0·27$\pm$ 0·28	5·21$\pm$1·04
Second	0·36$\pm$ 0·16	2·86$\pm$ 0·43	1·02$\pm$ 0·56	0·71$\pm$ 0·41	0·71$\pm$0·43	7·35$\pm$1·00
Third	0·25$\pm$ 0·016	4·29$\pm$ 3·04	0·55$\pm$ 0·38	0·94$\pm$ 0·36	0·22$\pm$0·04	4·65$\pm$0·48
Fourth	210·90$\pm$ 7·20	333·70$\pm$ 29·9	53·46$\pm$ 10·5	2·03$\pm$ 0·40	20·93$\pm$4·90	53·10$\pm$10·8
	129·10	54·20	—	—	—	21·00

[1] Animals received 50 mg thorium but for convenience of comparison the results are given for 25 mg

contact with the substance administered. This assumption is confirmed by histoautoradiography of these organs. The largest number of tracks was noted in the capsule and the subcapsular tissue. Therefore, it is quite possible that the true amount of thorium deposited in the tissues was within the range of values close to the content in the liver and spleen for rats of the second and third groups particularly since the thorium content of the other organs, with no possibility of contamination, was in general identical in the rats of the first three groups.

The highest concentration of thorium was found in the bone tissue* and then in the spleen. The amount of thorium found per 1 g of liver was approximately 20 times less than in bone tissue. Thorium was also found in the circulating blood.

On intracardiac injection of thorium citrate the distribution of thorium in the organs and tissues differed from that already indicated (Table 1). The highest concentration of thorium citrate was found in the liver and spleen. In the bone tissue and kidneys it was 4–6 times less and in the muscular tissue 10–15 times less while in the blood only traces of thorium were found.

As indicated above, on intracardiac injection of thorium nitrate only one rat survived. In it we investigated the thorium content of the liver, spleen and bone tissue. As Table 1 shows, the distribution of thorium in the organs of this rat was almost the same as after administration of thorium citrate.

In Table 2 the amount of thorium found in the intact organs and tissues is given as percentage of the total amount found in the animal body.

Table 2 shows that the results for the second and third groups are similar. In the bone tissue 53–75 per cent was found, in the liver and spleen only 1–3 per cent, in the blood about 3 per cent, in muscle tissue from 10–20 per cent while other organs and tissues accounted for 5–16 per cent. For the fourth group the percentage deposition differed considerably. In the bone tissue only 11 per cent was deposited, in the liver 17 per cent and in the spleen 3 per cent, in the kidneys 3 per cent, in muscle tissue 20 per cent and in the general blood 0·3 per cent. For the other organs and tissues the value was 44 per cent.

We were interested in the ratio between the amount of thorium administered and absorbed and also between the amount of thorium administered and its content in the individual organs and tissues; these findings are presented in Table 3.

* Despite the great practical and theoretical interest of the problem of the deposition of thorium in the bone marrow we were not able in our experiments to carry out this investigation since the amount of bone marrow in the long bones of rats is negligible and insufficient for analysis.

TABLE 2. *Content of Thorium in Whole Organ as Percentage of That Found in the Body*

Group	Route	Thorium administered	Chemical compound
First	Intraperitoneally	25 mg	Thorium nitrate
Second	Intramuscularly	25 mg	Thorium nitrate
Third	Orally[2]	25 mg	Thorium nitrate
Fourth	Intracardiac	25 mg	Thorium citrate complex

	Liver	Spleen	Kidneys	Blood[3]	Muscle[3]	Bone[3]	Other organs[4]
First	64·16 (1·69)[1]	6·52 (3·72)	0·18 (0·59)	2·52 (8·15)	4·43 (14·30)	19·01 (61·35)	3·15 (10·17)
Second	1·06	1·00	0·56	3·66	23·45	53·56	16·62
Third	1·75	2·94	0·83	3·03	10·67	75·14	5·60
Fourth	17·59	3·06	2·83	0·30	20·33	11·50	44·27

[1] Numerals in parentheses denote the distribution of thorium by organs on the assumption that the true concentration of thorium in the liver and spleen is considerably lower than that found and is approximately equal to that on intramuscular and oral administration.

[2] The animals received 50 g thorium, but for convenience of comparison the results are given for 25 mg.

[3] Total weight of such tissues as blood, muscle and bone are taken from the tables of Zakutinskii (1959).

[4] The concentrations of thorium in the muscles were used for calculating these findings.

Table 3 shows that an insignificant amount of thorium nitrate was absorbed from the site of administration. On entering the gastro-intestinal tract about 0·5 per cent was absorbed in 72 hr and in the contents of the intestines about 64 per cent of the amount administered was found. On intraperitoneal injection 0·9 per cent of the given dose was absorbed and on intramuscular 2 per cent. The remainder was retained for a long time at the site of administration. In view of the losses of thorium during preparation of the biological material before the thorium determination as can be seen from the last column of Table 3, it is difficult to judge the differences in absorption in the various groups. It may be supposed that for the different sites of entry not more than 2 per cent is absorbed. Thus, a large amount of thorium is deposited in the bones, between 0·4 and 0·7 per cent of the administered amount. In the liver and spleen the deposition is considerably less (40–50 times) than in the bone. On oral administration the values for the liver were even smaller—0·0099 per cent and for the spleen 0·0166 per cent.

On intracardiac injection different percentage ratios were found: in the liver 10·49, spleen 1·84, kidneys 1·69, blood 0·18, muscles 12·16, bone 6·86 and other organs 26·41 per cent.

TABLE 3. *Distribution of Thorium by Organs as Percentage of the Amount Administered*

Group	Route	Thorium introduced in mg	Chemical compound	Amount of thorium as % of amount introduced		
				Liver	Spleen	Kidneys
First	Intraperitoneally	25	Thorium nitrate	0·012	0·027	0·004
Second	Intramuscularly	25	Thorium nitrate	0·014	0·013	0·007
Third	Orally	50	Thorium nitrate	0·0099	0·016	0·0047
Fourth	Intracardiac	25	Thorium citrate complex	10·49	1·84	1·65

	Amount of thorium as % of amount introduced							
	Blood	Muscle	Bone	Other organs	Excreted in urine and faeces	Absorbed	Remaining at site administration	Total found
First	0·069	0·104	0·450	0·074	0·159	0·889	90·21	91·09
Second	0·049	0·318	0·726	0·226	0·732	2·085	90·95	93·03
Third	0·0171	0·0503	0·424	0·029	0·0077	0·559	63·05	63·61
Fourth	0·18	12·16	6·86	26·41	21·78	100·0	—	81·41

Table 4 presents the results for excretion of thorium in the urine and faeces in the 72 hr elapsing after administration of thorium nitrate and thorium citrate.

The table shows that in the rats of the first three groups the amount of thorium excreted in the urine was much less than that found in the faeces. Urinary excretion was small and did not depend on the amount or pathway of excretion of thorium. In the rats of the fourth group given an intracardiac injection of thorium citrate excretion occurred chiefly in the urine. The total amount excreted in three days in the rats of the first two groups was only 0·159 and 0·732 per cent of the dose given. On entry of thorium via the gastro-intestinal tract its total amount excreted from the body in the faeces was 63·05–63·61 per cent of that given or 99·01 per cent of the amount found whereas for intracardiac injection of thorium citrate about

21·78 per cent of the dose given was excreted in the urine. The ratio of thorium excreted in the urine and faeces varied within wide limits. In the rats of the first three groups it varied over the range 1:10–1:4000 as against the ratio of 7:1 in the fourth group.

The present paper does not give the results of histoautoradiography since, with a small content of thorium in organs and tissues, despite the lengthy exposure it was not possible to obtain reliable information on the content and distribution of thorium.

The material obtained by us is in the main in agreement with the findings of other workers: soluble thorium compounds introduced directly into the bloodstream accumulate chiefly in the liver but when administered by other routes in bone tissue. Our findings (Table 1) clearly show that after intraperitoneal and intramuscular injection and when introduced via the gastro-intestinal tract, the largest amount of thorium per gram tissue settles in the bones. This value corresponds to the deposition in all the skeleton of 53–75 per cent of the total amount detected in the organs and tissues. It is also clear that irrespective of the route of administration, the distribution and accumulation of thorium in individual organs and tissues are of the same order of magnitude. On administration of thorium directly into the bloodstream (in our case, intracardiac) the largest amount per gram tissue was found in the liver and spleen. For the same route of administration thorium nitrate and thorium citrate were distributed and deposited in the organs similarly. This confirms the legitimacy of comparing results obtained on intracardiac administration of thorium citrate with those for administration of thorium nitrate by other routes.

Thus, a certain pattern can be seen in the distribution of thorium for different routes of administration which one may attempt to explain on

TABLE 4. *Excretion of Thorium in Urine and Faeces (in 72 hr after Administration of its Nitrate and Citrate) as Percentage of the Amount Administered*

Group	Route	Thorium administered	Chemical compound	Urine	Faeces	Total excreted in urine and faeces	Ratio of excretion in urine and faeces
First	Intraperitoneally	25 mg	Thorium citrate	0·014	0·145	0·159	1 : 10
Second	Intramuscularly	25 mg	Thorium nitrate	0·010	0·722	0·732	1 : 70
Third	Orally	50 mg	Thorium nitrate	0·015	63·61	63·625	1 : 4240
Fourth	Intracardiac	25 mg	Thorium citrate	18·96	2·82	21·78	7 : 1

the basis of the physicochemical and biological mechanisms of absorption, accumulation and excretion of chemical elements in the body. According to the available evidence, the behaviour of chemical elements in the body is determined by their chemical and physicochemical properties (Zakutinskii 1959; Tarusov, 1954; Balabukha and Fradkin, 1958).

An element on entering the body enters into reactions with the different body components, tissue fluids, plasma, cells. As a result, readily soluble and completely dissociated or poorly soluble and poorly dissociating compounds form. Depending on this the substances may be in the body in the form of free ions or colloids. Elements in the ionic state mostly accumulate in the bone tissue and in the colloidal form in the liver, spleen and bone marrow. But this does not exclude the possible accumulation of colloids in the bone tissue too, because this depends on the degree of their dispersion (Zakutinskii, 1959). In our work, thorium, a tetravalent heavy metal, has the properties of a high valency and is able to form complexes. It is also known that it is heavily hydrolysed in media with pH above 3·5. The hydroxide forms chainlike complexes and behaves as a colloid very poorly soluble in water. Its solubility product at 25°C is 10^{-39}. It dissolves well only in solutions with which it complexes—solutions of carbonates, citrates and tartrates (Katz and Seaborg, 1957).

Examination of our findings in the light of the above remarks explains the negligibly small absorption of thorium from the site of administration and the character of its distribution in the organs and tissues. There is no doubt that any soluble thorium compound on entry into the body will be heavily hydrolysed since the pH of the body is higher than 3·5. As pointed out by Zakutinskii (1959) and Tarusov (1954), absorption is directly related to the degree of hydrolysis of the substance. This means that on intraperitoneal and intramuscular injection thorium will be poorly absorbed, i.e. a large part of it will remain at the site of administration while on oral administration it will be excreted from the body in the faeces. From the fact that accumulation chiefly occurs in the bone tissue for these routes of administration, it may be indirectly concluded that thorium enters the bloodstream either in the form of an ion or in the form of a finely dispersed colloid. After intracardiac administration where accumulation is predominantly in the liver and spleen, the chemistry of the solutions formed is very complex (McClinton and Schubert, 1948). The thorium may be in the form of ions and finely dispersed colloids, but chiefly in the form of coarsely dispersed colloids or colloid-like particles. Evidence of the validity of our assumption is also provided by excretion of thorium in the urine. Since renal filtration and active excretion are in fact primarily determined by the size of the excreted particles (Dobson *et al.*, 1949) it becomes clear why for the first three routes of administration the amount excreted is negligible (which is connected with the minimum absorption of thorium) while it is higher for the intracardiac route. In the latter case this is to be explained by the instant penetration into the bloodstream of a large amount of thorium in a form readily diffusing free ions of thorium, or thorium citrate.*

In confirmation of this we may invoke the results obtained by Boone *et al.* (1958). Their experiments with ionium (thorium^{230}) in rats are in agreement with ours, the only difference being that the thorium excreted was determined for 24 hr. The results show that the largest amount of thorium is found during the first 24 hr in the urine. Excretion in the faeces is negligible during this period. On subsequent days excretion in the urine becomes considerably lower than the amount excreted in the faeces.

So far it has been impossible to give a definite explanation of the mechanism of excretion of thorium in the faeces. Naturally, the idea of biliary elimination arises or excretion through the mucosa of the large intestine similar to lead and other heavy metals. However, this idea requires special verification.

Summary

1. After intraperitoneal, intramuscular and oral administration between 53 and 75 per cent of the amount of thorium found in the body is in the bone tissue. The amount in other organs and tissues is much less and the amount in the whole body does not exceed 2 per cent of that administered.

2. On intracardiac administration of thorium citrate and thorium nitrate the thorium mainly accumulates in the liver (17 per cent) and spleen (3 per cent).

3. During the first three days following intraperitoneal and intramuscular injection of thorium nitrate only 0·159–0·732 per cent of the amount administered is excreted in the urine and faeces. The excretion in the urine varies from 0·01 to 0·015 per cent of the amount administered and does not depend on the route of administration.

4. During the first three days following intracardiac administration of thorium citrate about 22 per cent of the amount administered is excreted, 19 per cent of this amount in the urine.

5. Apparently, absorption, distribution and excretion of thorium on intraperitoneal, intramuscular and oral administration have common physicochemical and biological mechanisms. On intracardiac administration there are certain special features in the distribution of thorium associated with the degree of dispersion of its compounds.

* In this case we speak only of thorium citrate because we were unable to collect urine from the rats given intracardiac thorium nitrate and we do not know whether excretion is the same for administration of these two thorium compounds.

References

ACKERMAN H. R., ALLEN P., BONNER G., DOWNS W. L., HODGE H. C., MAYNARD E. A., NEUMAN W. F., SCOTT J. K., SPARKS A. and STOCKINGER H. E., Preliminary Studies of the Toxicity of Thorium. AECD-2283 (UR-13) (1948).

BALABUKHA V. S. and FRADKIN G. YE., *Accumulation of Radioactive Elements in the Body and Their Elimination (Nakopleniye radioaktivnykh elementov v organizme i ikh vyvedeniye)*. Medgiz (1958).

BOONE I. U., ROGERS B. S., WHITE D. C. and HARRIS P. S., Toxicity, Excretion and Tissue Distribution of Ionium (Th^{230}) in Rats. *Amer. Industr. Hyg. Ass.* **19**, 4, 285–295 (1958).

DOBSON E. L., GOFMAN J. W., JONES H. B., KELLY L. S. and WALKER L. A., Studies with Colloids containing Radioisotopes of Yttrium, Zirconium, Columbium and Lanthanum. *J. Lab. clin. Med.* **34**, 3, 305–312 (1949).

ERLEKSOVA YE., V., *Distribution of Certain Radioactive Elements in Animals (Raspredeleniye nekotorykh radioaktivnykh elementov v organizme zhivotnykh)*. Medgiz (1960).

KATZ J. J. and SEABORG G. T. *The Chemistry of the Actinide Elements*, Methuen & Co. Ltd., London (1957).

KUZNETSOV V. I. and SAVVIN S. V., Sensitive Photometric Determination of Thorium with the Arsenazo-3 Reagent (Chustvitel'noye fotometricheskoye opredeleniye toriya s reagentom arsenazoi-3). *Radiokhimiya* **III**, 1, 79–86 (1961).

MCCLINTON L. T. and SCHUBERT J., Toxicity of Some Zirconium and Thorium Salts in Rats. *J. Pharmacol. Exp. Ther.* **94**, 1–6 (1948).

SALERNO P. R. and MATTIS P. A., Absorption and Distribution of Thorium Nitrate in the Rat. *J. Pharmacol. Exp. Ther.* **101**, 31–32 (1951).

SCHUBERT J., FINKE M., WHITE M. and HIRSCH G., Plutonium and Yttrium Content of the Blood, Liver and Skeleton of the Rat at Different Times after Intravenous Administration. *Biol. Chem.* **182**, 2, 635–642 (1950).

SCOTT J. K., NEUMAN W. F. and BONNER J. F., The Distribution and Excretion of Thorium Sulphate. *J. Pharmacol. Exp. Ther.* **106**, 296–290 (1952).

TARUSOV B. N., *Bases of the Biological Effect of Radioactive Emanations (Osnovy biologichsekogo deistviya radioaktivnykh izluchenii)*. Medgiz (1954).

THOMAS R. G., The Metabolism of Thorium 230 (Ionium) Administered by Intratracheal Injection to the Rat. UR-480 (1956).

YAN SYAO-SHAN, Toxicology of Thorium (Materialy po toksikologii toriya). Dissertation, Moscow (1962).

YAN SYAO-SHAN, Behaviour of Thorium Dioxide in Rats on Intratracheal Administration (Povedeniye dvuokisi toriya v organizme krys pri intratrakheal'nom vvedenii). *Gig. trud. i profzabolevan.* **6**, 10, 46–51 (1962).

ZAKUTINSKII D. I., *Aspects of Toxicology of Radioactive Substances (Voprosy toksikologii radioaktivnykh veshchestv)*. Medgiz (1959).

ZAKUTINSKII D. I., PARFENOV YU. D. and SELIVANOVA L. N., *Reference Book on the Toxicology of Radioactive Isotopes (Spravochnik po toksikologii radioaktivnykh izotopov)*. Medgiz (1962).

THE BEHAVIOUR OF THORIUM DIOXIDE IN RATS AFTER INTRATRACHEAL AND INTRAPERITONEAL ADMINISTRATION

YAN SYAO-SHAN

THORIUM-232 is an alpha emitter with a long half-life ($1{\cdot}39 \times 10^{10}$ years) and therefore its deposition in the body may be a danger to health. The behaviour of thorium dioxide in the body on entry into the lungs has been little studied so that it is not possible to make a proper assessment of the degree of its radiotoxicity.

Studies have been reported in the literature concerning the fate of certain thorium compounds after entry into the body via the respiratory tract. Thus, Scott *et al.*, (1952) noted that after inhalation of thorium compounds the bulk was found in the lungs with only an insignificant amount in other organs.

Frolova (1959), systematically studying the behaviour of thorium fluoride given to the animals intratracheally, found thorium was mainly deposited in the lungs and trachea during 80 days' observation. However, thorium was found in the sternum, spleen, blood and lymph nodes during the first ten days. In 80 days' observation thorium was not found either in the liver or kidneys, nor was it found in the urine. During the first 7 to 8 days after administration, 4–31·5 per cent of the dose given was excreted in the faeces. Frolova gives no information on the behaviour of thorium at later stages.

Tarasenko (1960) studied the behaviour of thorium fluoride for a considerable time after intratracheal administration (120 days). Together with the above-indicated localizations of thorium the author found it to be present in bone, brain, muscles, heart and kidneys. The highest radioactivity was recorded in the lungs, trachea and bone. The presence of thorium in other organs was attributed by Tarasenko to the fact that thorium introduced into the lung undergoes partial solution and enters the blood.

Albert (1955) as a result of examination of workers in plant refining thorium from monazite presented information on chronic deposition of thorium in the lungs.

Hodge (1960) considering that short period inhalation of thorium does not produce reliable signs of intoxication carried out an experiment in which animals (dogs, rats) were daily exposed by inhalation for one year. Thorium was detected in the lungs, liver, kidneys, spleen and bones. Accumulation of thorium in the lungs increased with the duration of exposure. After one year exposure the amount of thorium in the lungs was five times greater than at the end of the first month. All these findings show that thorium after entering the lung via the respiratory tract is poorly eliminated and retained for a long time at the site of introduction.

The published findings mentioned provide a definite idea of the behaviour of thorium compounds in the body. Nevertheless, this problem cannot be considered completely solved. The distribution of thorium in the body is primarily influenced by the route of administration and also by the degree of its solubility in biological media. The behaviour in the body of poorly soluble thorium compounds following intratracheal administration will differ from that described by many workers for other modes of administration (subcutaneous, intravenous, intraperitoneal, etc.). And although inhalation is the most realistic one for contact with thorium in industry this problem has still received little study. In addition, methods of investigation of the content of thorium in biological media used by many authors are insufficiently sensitive to judge the quantitative ratios of thorium in different organs which is of great importance for establishing health standards.

Parenterally administered thorium is retained for a long time in the body and its absorption from the site of administration is very low. The work of Amory (1948), Vögtlin and Minder (1952), Vakhtel' (1957), Budin and Gershon-Cohen (1956) and others, has demonstrated the presence of Thorotrast in the kidneys after pyelography, in the brain after cerebral arteriography, in the tissue of the mammary glands after mammography and in the cavity of the lesser pelvis after salpingography. Eighteen years after intraperitoneal injection of Thorotrast, thorium was localized in connective tissue and in the serous membrane of the organs and walls of the abdominal cavity. It was also found in the perirenal cellular tissue. On administration of Thorotrast directly in the ventricles of the brain, thorium persisted for a long time (33 months) in the sub-arachnoid and perivascular spaces of the brain.

Lyass (1960) described four cases in which Thorotrast was found for 6–9 years in the soft tissues of the neck after unsuccessful cerebral angiography. The radioactivity of the solid infiltrate in the neck produced a considerable absorbed radiation dose while the ThO_2 remained there.

The results of clinical observations and experimental investigations of other authors showed that the main sites of deposition of thorium after intraperitoneal administration of Thorotrast are the omentum, mesenterium, aponeurosis of the abdominal wall, diaphragm and lymph nodes

(Efskind, 1940; Lindenbraten, 1950; Hale, 1953; and others). Thus, Efskind injected rabbits intraperitoneally with 5 ml Thorotrast (25 per cent colloidal solution of thorium dioxide) and found that the substance deposited in the first place in the omentum, mesenterium, the linea alba and the diaphragm. These accumulations were found chiefly in the subperitoneal connective tissue, mainly in the phagocytes, and their amount did not change during 6 months' observation.

Intraperitoneally injected Thorotrast is eliminated from the abdominal cavity very slowly. Lindenbraten (1950) reported that after introduction of Thorotrast into the peritoneum, in the first 15–30 min the substance located close to the diaphragm rapidly passed into the lymphatics of the

TABLE 1. *Size of Thorium Dioxide Particles in μ*

Sample No.	Number of ThO_2 particles						
	Under 2	2–4	4–6	6–8	8–10	Over 10	Total in sample
1	4	166	28	1	1	0	200
2	5	147	46	2	0	0	200
3	4	160	32	4	0	0	200
Total (absolute number)	13	473	106	7	1	0	600
% of total particle count	2·16	78·78	17·68	1·17	0·17	0	100

anterior chest wall and from there into the network of fine lymphatics and the lymph nodes. Subsequently, the thorium dioxide coagulated and most of it gradually passed into the greater omentum and subphrenic space.

Thus, according to published findings thorium dioxide injected intraperitoneally is virtually not excreted from the body.

We studied the behaviour of thorium dioxide in the body after intratracheal administration. In the literature there are indications that dispersion of dust influences its fate in the respiratory tract. This equally applies to radioactive aerosols, especially alpha emitters. From the point of view of the radiological danger, the particle size of alpha emitters acquires special importance. It is well known that the total area of the surface of dust particles for the same gravimetric amount depends on particle size. In view of the major influence of the size of dust particles on their behaviour in the body and the intensity of damage to the surrounding tissue, we determined the dispersion of thorium dioxide.

The size of the particles of thorium dioxide dust was determined by the standard method using ocular and objective micrometers. The results of the measurements are given in Table 1.

As Table 1 shows, the suspension of thorium dioxide administered contained 80·9 per cent particles with a size up to 4 μ which on inspiration may penetrate into the deep sections of the lungs and be retained there.

Thorium dioxide was used in three series of experiments carried out on 36 adult male white rats weighing 200–250 g. Each of the series was divided into groups depending on the time of determination after administration of thorium dioxide (first series) or the dose of thorium (second series).

In the first series of experiments (20 rats) we studied the excretion and the distribution of thorium in the organs and tissues of rats at 1, 3, 5, 7 and 10 days and 5 and 21 months after intratracheal administration of 20 mg of thorium dioxide per kg of rat weight (5 mg pure thorium per kg rat weight).

The animals of the second series (10 rats) were injected intratracheally with thorium dioxide in amounts of 2, 20, 200, 300 and 400 mg/kg body weight. The rats were killed after 13 months and the amount of thorium was determined in their organs and tissues by histoautoradiography.

The third series of experiments (3 rats) was carried out in order to establish the period of time for which the thorium dioxide remained at the site of injection. The rats were injected intraperitoneally with 600 mg of thorium dioxide per kg of body weight. The amount of thorium dioxide remaining at the site of administration after 15 months was measured. In all the experiments the total volume of suspension of thorium dioxide injected in saline did not exceed 1 ml.

Intratracheal administration of thorium dioxide was carried out by the bloodless method described by Gorodenskaya (1951) as modified by Levina and Gorbachevskaya (1955). Quantitative determination of thorium in the biosubstrates was made by a method proposed for ores by Kuznetsova and Savvin (1961) and modified for biosubstrates by Pavlovskaya and Cherkashina (this volume). The method is based on the formation of complex compounds of thorium with arsenazo-3. This compound depending on concentration is pink to emerald-green. The sensitivity of the method is 0·1 in 5 ml solution and the error of determination does not exceed 10 per cent.

To measure the content of thorium in the rat organs after administration of thorium dioxide it was found necessary to determine the natural content of thorium in the body. According to the findings reported by Voinar (1960) the human and animal body contains about 10^{-7} g thorium per 100 g fresh tissue. We know of no specific information on the content of thorium in the rat body. Therefore, for this purpose we determined the natural content in organs of normal rats but despite the high sensitivity of the method used by us no thorium was found in the organs of normal rats. Different results were obtained in experiments on rats given thorium dioxide. As Table 2 shows, 5 days after intratracheal administration of thorium dioxide, thorium was found in nearly all the organs and tissues of the rats. At later times it was determined only in the lungs, trachea, the lymph nodes of the portals of the lungs, cervical nodes and in the bones. In other organs, the content of thorium fell and with time disappeared.

Most of the intratracheally administered thorium dioxide was retained in the lungs. In the first 24 hr, 68–73 per cent of the amount given was found there. The fall in the content occurred very slowly and even after 21 months 15–30 per cent of the thorium administered was still found in the lungs. The prolonged retention of thorium dioxide in the lungs may be explained by the negligible solubility of thorium in plasma (Bokova, 1960) and furthermore the small fraction which dissolves undergoes hydrolysis with the formation of the poorly soluble thorium hydroxide which precipitates.

In the lymph nodes (bifurcation and cervical), thorium was found in considerable amounts (1–2 per cent of that administered) during the first few days. At late times the content of thorium fell. It is clear that after introduction into the lung a small part of the thorium dioxide enters the lymph nodes via the lymphatics, where it is retained for a long time. During the first days after administration thorium was found in the circulating blood and urine. Apparently, in the initial stages, there is activation of phagocytic reactions aimed at clearing the lungs of particles of thorium oxide. Subsequently, corresponding to the reduction in the content of thorium in the circulating blood, there is an increase in the amount in the liver, spleen and bone marrow, which indicates the tropism of thorium for organs rich in reticulo-endothelial elements. A considerable amount of thorium was excreted in the faeces in the first few days after administration; in the first day 6–8 per cent was excreted and in 5 days 9–14 per cent of the amount administered. Excretion in the faeces occurred probably through swallowing particles of thorium dioxide which had moved up from the mucosa of the trachea and bronchi. At late times, thorium was found in 24 hr faeces samples irregularly and in insignificant amounts.

As indicated above, to study retention of thorium at the site of administration, its behaviour and late sequelae, the rats were given intraperitoneally thorium dioxide in an amount of 600 mg/kg body weight. Three rats were killed 15 months after administration to determine the thorium content of the organs of the abdominal cavity and the amount in the femoral bone. Autopsy of the animals revealed accumulations of thorium oxide under the serous membrane of the organs of the abdominal cavity. Since

TABLE 2. *Content of* ThO_2 *in Organs and Excreta of Rats at Various Times after Intratracheal Injection (as Percentage of the Dose Administered)*

Organ or tissue	Times after administration						
	1 day	3 days	5 days	7 days	10 days	5 months	21 months
Lungs and trachea	68–73	65–70	64–72	60–70	50–65	25–40	15–30
Bifurcation and cervical lymph nodes	1–2	1–2	1–2	0·8–1	0·7–1·0	0–0·2	Traces
Gastro-intestinal tract plus contents	3–5	2–3·5	0·5–1·0	0–0·4	Traces	0–0·25	0
Liver	0·1–0·4	0·3–0·6	0–0·3	0·1–0·3	0–0·3	0–0·1	0
Spleen	0–0·2	0·1–0·2	0·1–0·3	0–0·17	0–0·1	0–Traces	0
Blood	0·1–1·0	0·7–1·3	0–0·83	0–Traces	0	0	0
Bone	0–0·8	1–2	0–3·5	3–6·5	3–5·5	2–4·7	3–2
Kidneys	0–0·1	0–0·3	0–Traces	0–Traces	0	0	0
Urine	0·3–0·5	0·2–0·6	0–0·5	0–Traces	0	0	0
Faeces	6–8	2–4	1–2	0–1	0	0–1·0	0·2

it was impossible to determine separately the amount of thorium in these accumulations on the surface and in the tissues of the organ, the organs were investigated as a whole. The findings obtained on their thorium level are presented in Table 3.

TABLE 3. *Content of Thorium in Organs of Abdominal Cavity and in Bones after Intraperitoneal Administration (as Percentage of the Dose Administered)*

Organ	Contents
Intestine	11–66·3
Liver, spleen	3·4–8·3
Femur	0·33–0·51

Thus, at late times a large amount of the administered thorium oxide remains at the site of administration. The presence of thorium in the femur indicates that a small amount of its dioxide is evidently dissolved and with passage of time deposited in bone.

In the third series of experiments the rats (2 per dose) were killed 13 months after intratracheal administration of thorium dioxide in amounts of 2, 20, 200, 300 and 400 mg/kg. The organs of these animals were investigated by histoautoradiography as described by Erleksova. In all the histoautoradiograms of the lungs and lymph nodes accumulations of particles were detected by alpha tracks from the thorium. For illlustration we give the histoautoradiograms of some rats (Figs. 1, 2, 3 and 4).

Figures 1–3 are the histoautoradiograms of the lungs of rats killed 13 months after intratracheal administration of various amounts of ThO_2 (2, 20, 300 mg/kg weight). In the lungs accumulations of thorium dioxide were seen. The tracks of alpha particles in the form of black dots (star shaped) are readily seen originating in the walls and cavities of the alveoli.

These histoautoradiograms show that the density of the accumulations of thorium oxide in the rat lungs differed with the amount administered, differences confirmed by the calculation of the density and size of the accu-

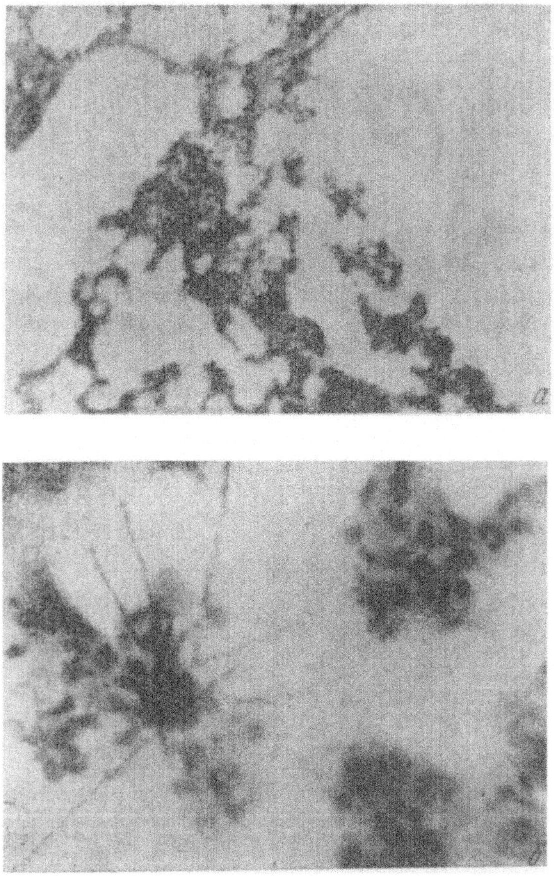

FIG. 1. Histoautoradiogram of lung tissue from rat No. 16 given 2 mg/kg ThO_2 intratracheally. Exposure 12 days. Staining with haematoxylin-eosin. (a) low magnification: ocular ×10, objective ×8, photographic enlargement ×3; (b) high magnification: ocular ×10, objective ×40, photographic enlargement ×3

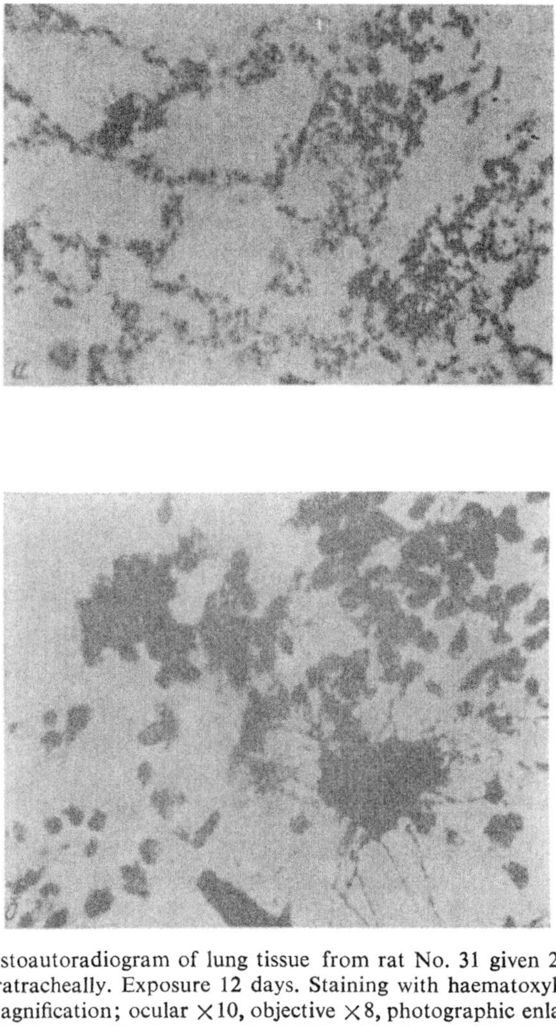

FIG. 2. Histoautoradiogram of lung tissue from rat No. 31 given 20 mg/kg ThO_2 intratracheally. Exposure 12 days. Staining with haematoxylin-eosin. (a) low magnification; ocular $\times 10$, objective $\times 8$, photographic enlargement $\times 3$; (b) high magnification: ocular $\times 10$, objective $\times 40$; photographic enlargement $\times 3$

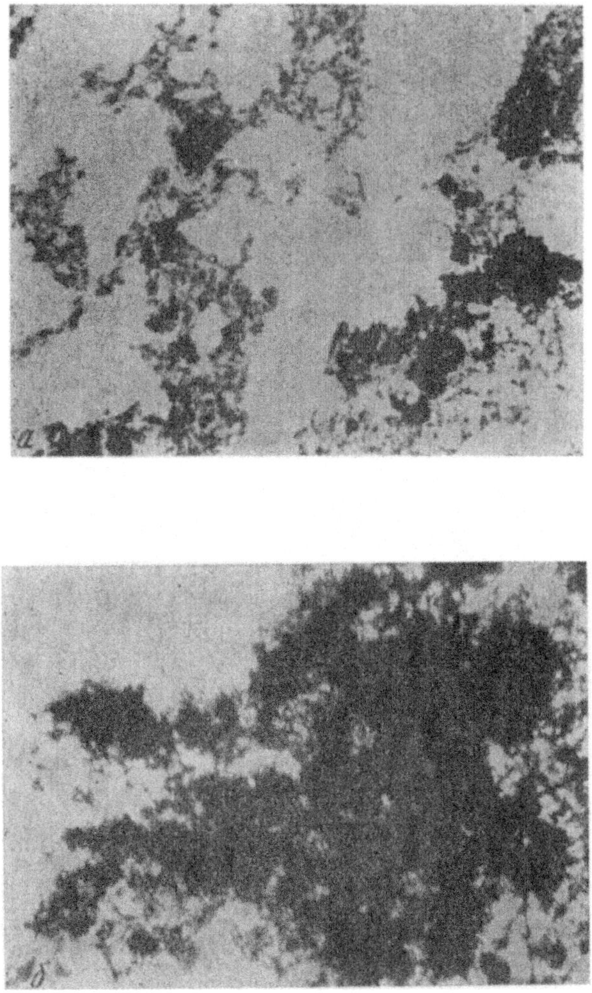

FIG. 3. Histoautoradiogram of lung tissue from rat No. 97 given 300 mg/kg ThO_2 intratracheally. Exposure for 12 days. Staining with haematoxylin-eosin. (a) low magnification: ocular ×10; objective ×8; photographic enlargement ×3; (b) high magnification: ocular ×10, objective ×10; photographic enlargement ×3

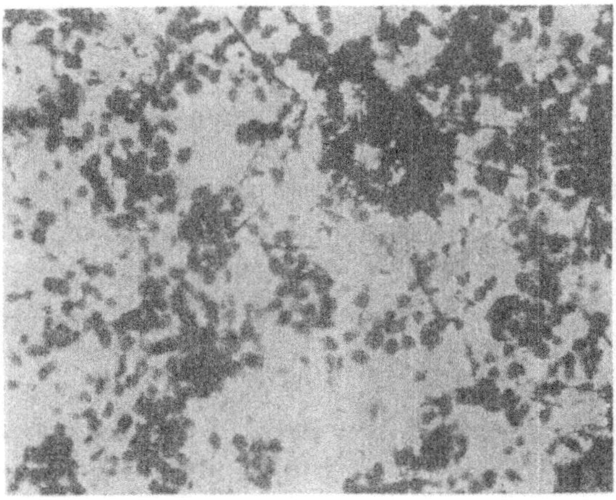

FIG. 4. Histoautoradiogram of cervical lymph node tissue from rat No. 97 receiving 300 mg/kg ThO_2 intratracheally. Exposure for 12 days. Staining with haematoxylin-eosin. Magnification: ocular ×10, objective ×40, photographic enlargement ×3

TABLE 4. *Density and Size of Accumulations of Thorium Dioxide in Lungs in Histoautoradiograms*

Rat No.	16	21	56	97
Dose of ThO_2 in mg/kg body weight	2	20	200	300
Density of accumulations in number of units per mm^2 lung tissue	0·8	9·5	82·7	89·6
Size of accumulations in m×m	8·6×11·5	11·5×14·4	17×20	144×345 (10% of all accumulations 37×37 (63%)

mulations of thorium oxide on microscopic inspection of the histoautoradiograms. The results obtained are given in Table 4.

Figure 4 shows the histoautoradiogram of the cervical lymph node tissues from rat No. 97. The alpha particle tracks of thorium in the lymphoid tissue are distinctly visible.

In histoautoradiograms of other organs no traces of thorium could be found.

Summary

1. In the first days (up to 5) after intratracheal administration thorium dioxide is found in the lungs, trachea, bifurcation and cervical lymph nodes, the gastro-intestinal tract and contents, liver, bones and kidney.

2. The largest amount of thorium was found in the lungs and in the early stages after administration this was 68–73 per cent of the dose given. After 21 months the rat lungs still contained 15–30 per cent of the thorium administered, which indicates the prolonged retention of thorium dioxide in the lungs. This was also confirmed by histoautoradiography.

3. Histoautoradiography of the lymph nodes of rats 13 months after intratracheal administration of thorium oxide showed accumulation of thorium, and alpha particle tracks were seen in lymphoid tissue.

4. Excretion of thorium dioxide in the urine and faeces was insignificant at late times after its intratracheal administration.

5. Following intraperitoneal administration thorium dioxide is retained for a long time in the abdominal cavity. After 15 months 14·4–74·6 per cent of the amount administered was found in the abdominal cavity and 0·33–0·51 per cent was found in the femoral bone.

References

Albert R., Klevin P., Fresco J., Harley J. S., Harris W. and Eisenbud M., Industrial Hygiene and Medical Survey of Thorium Refinery, *Arch. ind. Health* **11**, 234–242 (1955).

Amory H. I. and Bunch R. F., Perivascular Injection of Thorotrast and Its Sequelae. *Radiology* **51**, 831–839 (1948).

Bokova G. B., Study of Behaviour with Time of Metallic Thorium and Some of Its Compounds (Izucheniye povedeniya metallicheskogo toriya i mekotorykh ego soyedenni v razlichnye sroki). *Gig. trud. i profzabolevan.* **1**, 49 (1960).

Budin E. and Gershon-Cohen J., The Danger of Cancer from Thorotrast as a Diagnostic Medium. *Amer. J. Roentgen.*, **75**, 1188 (1956).

Efskind L., Örtliche Veränderungen bei intraperitonealer Injection von Thorium dioxyd (Thorotrast). *Acta Chirurgica Scandinavica* **84**, 79–85 (1940).

Frolova I. A., Distribution and Elimination of Thorium in Rats on Intratracheal Administration of Its Insoluble Salts (Raspredeleniye ivyvedeniye toriya u krys pri intratrakheal'nom vvedenii ego nerastvorimoi soli). *1957 Collection of Abstracts on Radiation Medicine (Sbornik reefratov po radiatsionnoi meditsine za 1957g)*. Vol. 1, pp. 131–132. Medgiz (1959).

Gorodenskaya Ye. N., Role of Colloidal Silicon Dioxide in the Mechanism of Genesis of Silicosis. (Rol' kolloidnoi dvuokisi kremniya v mekhanizme vozniknoveniya silikoza). In: *Silicosis (Silikoz)*. Moscow (1951).

Hale A. R. and Baillif R. N., The Retention and Elimination of Colloidal Thorium Dioxide in Albino Rat following Protracted Administration. *Anat. Rec.* **117**, 2, 163–176 (1953).

Hodge H. C., Maynard E. A. and Leach L. J., The Chemical Toxicity of Thorium Dioxide following Inhalation by Laboratory Animals. University of Rochester N.Y. Report UR-562 (1960).

KUZNETSOVA V. I. and SAVVIN S. V., Sensitive Photometric Determination of Thorium with the Reagent Arsenazo III. *Radiokhimiya* III, 1, 79–86 (1961).

LEVINA E. I. and GORBACHEVSKAYA YE. G., Changes in Lung Tissue on Intratracheal Administration of Manganese Oxides (Izmenenie legochnoi tkani pri vnutritrakheal'nom vvedeniya oksilov margantsa). *Gig. i. sanitar.* **1**, 25–28 (1955).

LYASS F. M., Late Complication after Diagnostic Use of a Long -lived Radioactive Substance (Thorium) (O pozdem oslozhnenii posle diagnosticheskogo primeneniya dolgozhivushchego radioaktivnogo veschestva (toriya). *Meditsinskaya radiologiya* **3**, 23–26 (1960).

PAVLOVSKAYA N. A. and CHERKASHINA T. N., This volume, pp. 83–86.

SCOTT J. K., NEUMAN W. F. and BONNER J. F., The Distribution and Excretion of Thorium Sulphate. *J. Pharmacol. Exp. Ther.* **106**, 286–290 (1952).

TARASENKO N. YU., Problem of the Toxicity of Thorium (K voprosu o toksichnosti toriya.) *Gig. trud. i profzabolevan.* **6**, 21–27 (1960).

VÖGTLIN J. and MINDER W., Über Thorotrastschäden nach Bronchographie, retrograder Pyelographie, Salpingographie und Arteriographie. *Radiol. clin.* **21**, 96, (1952).

VOINAR A. I., Quantitative Content of Trace Elements in the Animal Body (Kolichestvennoye soderzhaniye mikroelementov v zhivotnom organizme). In: *Biological Role of Trace Elements in the Animal and Human Body (Biologichskaya rol' mikroelementov v organizme zhivotnykh i cheloveka)*. Vysshei shkoly, Moscow (1960).

THE EFFECT OF THORIUM DIOXIDE ON THE PERIPHERAL BLOOD OF RATS

YAN SYAO-SHAN

THE absence of information on the toxicity of Thorotrast led to the wide introduction of colloidal thorium dioxide in medical practice in radio diagnosis. In the first years of its application there were no reports in the literature on the harmful effect of Thorotrast. Thus, in clinical use with usual doses of thorium (75 ml Thorotrast containing 15 g metallic thorium for hepatolienography, 30 ml Thorotrast for arteriography or bronchiography), in the early stages after its administration its toxicity was barely apparent (Looney, 1960). The immediate reaction to intravasal administration of Thorotrast consisted in transient fever, headaches, nausea, temporary anaemia, leucopenia and lymphocytosis. Petechiae rarely appeared. All these manifestations were short-lived, irregular and usually noted quite seldom (Thomas *et al.*, 1951).

Nevertheless, the published material entitles us to speak of the effect of thorium (Thorotrast) on the haemopoietic system. Thus, there are indications that anaemia, leukaemia and panmyelopathies appear at late stages after administration of Thorotrast. Lambin and Gerard (1932), Gottlieb (1933), Spier *et al.* (1947) and Duane (1957) reported on the appearance of aplastic or hypoplastic anaemia in persons after intravasal administration of Thorotrast for diagnostic purposes. Spier described one case of aplastic anaemia in a patient which appeared nine years after intravenous injection of Thorotrast for the purpose of hepatolienography. Analysis of the blood showed haemoglobin 3 g, erythrocytes 1,260,000 per mm^3, hypochromatosis, poikilocytosis and anisocytosis of the erythrocytes with a white cell count of 450–950 per mm^3 and differential count: lymphocytes 88 per cent, segmented nuclear neutrophils 2 per cent, rod nuclear neutrophils 1 per cent, juvenile cells 8 per cent and basophils 1 per cent. The haematocrit stood at 8 per cent. As was established at autopsy, aplasia of the haemopoietic tissue was the cause of death. In determining thorium in the organs of the deceased the author found it to be present in the bone marrow and spleen.

A similar case was also described by Duane (1957). The aplastic anaemia appeared in the patient 14 years after hepatolienography in which 75 ml of Thorotrast was administered. The radioactivity administered in terms of alpha radiation was the equivalent to 1·4 mg radium. On radioscopy the authors found accumulation of thorium in the liver and spleen. For purposes of therapy Duane attempted to stimulate excretion of Thorotrast from the body of the patient with an EDTA preparation but failed. Between 8 and 9 years after cerebral arteriography Grote and Pampas (1955) found leucopenia and neutropenia in one patient. Intravenous injection of thorium dioxide (Montanari-Reggiani *et al.*, 1933) led in rabbits and rats at first to leucopenia and at late stages to prolonged leucocytosis. Weil and Menefrier (1937) proposed that erythraemia be treated with thorium X—one of the radioactive daughters of thorium which is an alpha emitter. Describing the advantage of this method for depressing haemopoiesis, the author emphasized that its use required extreme caution since it may lead to severe late sequelae. Bone marrow insufficiency as a result of intravenous injection of Thorotrast has been described by Hieronymi and Sandkühler (1957). Netoušek *et al.* (1957) reported on a case of chronic myelosis developing 23 years after hepatolienography using Thorotrast. Analysis of the bone marrow showed that the granuloblasts in it accounted for 89 per cent of the total number of nucleated cells. Thorium dioxide was found in the reticular cells of the bone marrow. Panmyelopathies in similar cases were described by Moeschlin *et al.* (1953) and Grebe (1954). Myeloid leukaemia was found by Gebauer and Heinecker (1955).

However, despite the considerable evidence pointing to involvement of haemopoiesis there is no unanimity of opinion on the effect on it of Thorotrast. Some workers consider that the haemopoietic system changes little with clinical use of Thorotrast. Thus, Backer (1956) made repeated analyses of peripheral blood in 222 patients between 3·2 and 19·1 years after administration of Thorotrast for encephalography. As controls he also investigated the blood in 236 normal subjects and 124 patients with the same diseases but who had never received Thorotrast. He found no appreciable differences in the blood picture in the patients who had and had not received Thorotrast.

There is little data in the literature on the effect of various thorium compounds on entering the body. Thus, Tarasenko (1960) studying the effect of thorium fluoride on repeated oral administration to rabbits found in the first months leucocytosis and a slight fall in red cell count of the peripheral blood. Then, these indices returned to the initial level. Insignificant changes were seen in the differential white cell count: reduction in the absolute number of segmented nuclear neutrophils and lymphocytes.

Mainx (1957) reported on cases of anaemia together with indistinct leucopenia (number of leucocytes between 4400 and 5000 per mm^3) in 18 of 38 workers handling luminous paints containing the daughter products of thorium decay—radiothorium and mesothorium.

From the published findings presented here it is clear that the effect of thorium on the blood system especially on intratracheal administration has been insufficiently studied. Change in the processes of haemopoiesis is one of the characteristic signs of the radiotoxic effect of radioactive substances. Therefore, in studying the toxicology of thorium dioxide we considered it necessary to investigate the state of the peripheral blood in rats in conditions of prolonged retention of ThO_2 in the lungs.

For this purpose all the test animals were divided into eight groups. The rats in the control (eighth) group numbered 30 with 20 in each of the seven test groups all given thorium dioxide. Rats of the first to fifth groups received single intratracheal injections of a suspension of thorium dioxide in saline in an amount of 2, 20, 200, 300 and 400 mg per kg body weight, or respectively $19{\cdot}2\times10^{-5}$, $19{\cdot}2\times10^{-4}$, $19{\cdot}2\times10^{-3}$, $29{\cdot}0\times10^{-3}$ and $38{\cdot}6\times10^{-3}$ μCi per kg. The suspension of thorium dioxide was injected intraperitoneally into the animals of the sixth and seventh groups in an amount of 1000 and 2400 mg per kg body weight, which in radioactivity was $96{\cdot}6\times10^{-3}$ and $23{\cdot}2\times10^{-2}$ μCi per kg weight. These amounts were roughly 0·25, 2·5, 25, 37, 50, 125 and 301 of the maximum permissible amounts of thorium for a single administration into the human lungs. The volume of the suspension per rat did not exceed 1 ml. In the control group the rats were treated intratracheally with saline in the same volume.

Intratracheal administration was carried out by the bloodless method described by us previously and intraperitoneal injection by the standard method. The duration of the observation was about 20 months.

Clinical signs of intoxication with thorium during the investigation were feebly marked. Immediately after intratracheal administration of thorium oxide the rats breathed with difficulty and had a severe cough. Two days later these signs disappeared and they were outwardly normal, they put on weight and only after 15–16 months was there a slight loss in weight but roughly within the same limits as in the control animals. At the end of the first year after administration the animals became listless and unkempt. Bald patches were seen in the majority of the test rats and the hair was dishevelled. We studied the change in the peripheral blood in the control animals and also in the test groups given thorium dioxide intratracheally in the amounts indicated above.

To assess the results we shall give certain published findings on the composition of the peripheral blood in white rats in normal conditions obtained by various authors (Table 1).

As Table 1 shows, all the indices of the peripheral blood according to the findings of different workers vary in rats within fairly wide limits.

TABLE 1. *The Composition of the Peripheral Blood of Normal White Rats Obtained by Various Authors*

Authors	Haemoglobin %	Erythrocytes in millions	Leucocytes in thousands	Lymphocytes %	Neutrophils %
P. P. Sakharov (1952	**105**	9·3	15·2	—	—
Kleinberger (quoted by P. P. Sakharov, 1952)	109–125	5·6–6·3	4·8–15·2	53·5–75	22–40
Baranski and Barkowa (1956)	96	8	9	70	22·3
K. R. Viktorov (1956)	110	6	15	67	30
D. Wirth (1956)	94·3	9·3	15·2	76·5	17·7
N. Shmeleva (1960)	—	—	19·4	81·7	14·9

On examination of 60 normal rats we obtained the following results (Table 2). For convenience of comparison in some columns the mean findings are presented as well as the limits of variation. As Tables 1 and 2 show, the results obtained by us are similar to those obtained by other workers. The reticulocyte count found by us coincides with that of Baranski and Barkowa (1956). According to these workers the mean number of reticulocytes in rats is 19‰ with variations from 5 to 31 per thousand.

TABLE 2. *The Composition of the Peripheral Blood of 60 Normal White Rats Obtained in the Author's Laboratory*

Haemoglobin %	Erythrocytes in millions	Leucocytes in thousands	Neutrophils %	Lymphocytes %	Eosinophils %	Basophils %	Monocytes %	Thrombocytes in thousands	Reticulocytes ‰
90–100	7·5–8·4	10·5–16·3	11·5–29 (20·7)	60–84·5 (73·6)	0·5–3	0–0·5	0–0·2	200–800	9–31 (16)

Red Blood

The number of erythrocytes, haemoglobin and the colour index in the great majority of test animals of all the groups did not differ from the corresponding indices in the controls throughout the observation period. The red cell count both in these and other rats varied on average from 7·5 to $8{\cdot}4 \times 10^6$, haemoglobin from 90 to 100 per cent and the colour index from

0·59 to 0·64. In individual animals burdened with thorium (in one rat of the second group and three rats of the fifth group) temporary anaemia was noted accompanied by sharp reticulocytosis. In a rat (No. 22) of the second group 14 months after administration of thorium dioxide the number of erythrocytes fell to 3·7 million, haemoglobin to 44 per cent with reticulocytosis reaching 359‰ while the white blood was within normal limits. These indices soon became normal again but after 2·5 months the rat died with intestinal haemorrhaging.

Three cases of anaemia of a similar character were observed in the fifth group a few days before death of the animals (lung abscess, cancer).

Although haemorrhaging was not established in the period of onset of anaemia, the character of the anaemia observed, high reticulocytosis up to 400‰, and the comparatively rapid restoration of the red cell count and haemoglobin, suggests the presence of an acute blood loss the causes of which might have been the ulceration of the intestinal mucosa and pulmonary haemorrhages found at autopsy of these animals.

We also observed some cases of anaemia of another character. In four animals of the third group shortly before death (cancer and lung abscess) there was fall in the number of erythrocytes to 6–5 million and haemoglobin to 60–70 per cent. Reticulocytosis was not observed. Wasting of the animals began in this period.

The number of reticulocytes in the blood in the rats of the first to fourth test groups varied within the same limits as in the control group, on average around 16‰ and only in the fifth group 3–6 months after administration of thorium was reticulopenia observed. In the rats of this group the number of reticulocytes three months after administration fell to $5{\cdot}6 + 0{\cdot}9$‰ and in the sixth month was $9{\cdot}3 + 1{\cdot}5$‰. Change in the mean numbers of reticulocytes during the chronic experiments is indicated in Fig. 1. In view of the similar values for the mean numbers of reticulocytes in the animals of the first four groups the figure presents the data for the three groups, control, third and fifth, which had the most marked reticulopenia.

Despite the lack of significance in the difference in the mean numbers of reticulocytes in animals of the third and fourth groups from those obtained in the controls, in the test groups of rats considerable scatter was observed in the variance series. However, there were no significant differences in the values of the variance coefficient (V) and σ in these groups of animals as compared with the controls.

In the animals of the fourth test group (300 mg of ThO_2 per kg of body weight) in some periods (1·5, 3, 6 and 8 months) after the start of the experiment there was a tendency for the reticulocyte count to rise and fall.

In order to satisfy ourselves of the significance of the difference in the distribution of reticulocytes in the animals of the fourth group as compared with the controls, these findings were treated by the χ^2 method. Table 3 presents the results of such treatment for the animals of the fourth group 1·5, 3, 6 and 8 months after administration of 300 mg of ThO_2 per kg of body weight and at the same times for the control group. In the latter most of the analyses (84 per cent) showed a reticulocyte count from 10 to 20‰, a very low number of analyses (2.5 per cent) indicated a reduced number of reticulocytes and finally, in 13·5 per cent of the cases the reticulocyte count was above 21‰.

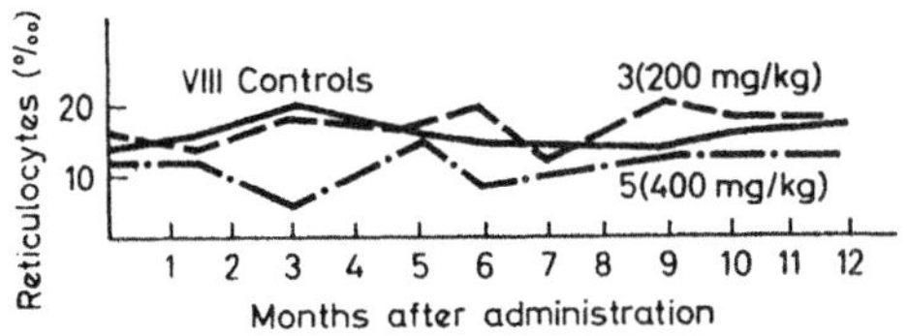

FIG. 1. Change in number of reticulocytes (‰) in rats after a single intratracheal administration of thorium dioxide

At the same times, in the fourth group 15·6 per cent of the analyses indicated a reduced number of reticulocytes and 25 per cent an increased number. The χ^2 value for this table was 13·85 which confirms the complete reliability of the material presented in the table (for a given value of χ^2 the null hypothesis is confirmed in less than 1 per cent of the cases).

TABLE 3. *Distribution of Reticulocytes in the Blood of Rats of the Fourth and Control Groups*

Group of rats	Total number of analyses	Analyses with reticulocyte count		
		Under 10 to 10‰	From 20‰	Over 20‰
Controls	37	2·5	84·0	13·5
Fourth	32	15·6	59·0	25·0

In the animals of the fifth group starting from 1·5 months after administration of 400 mg/kg ThO_2 and more so after 3 and 6 months, a considerable number of cases of reticulopenia was observed with reticulocyte count 9‰ and lower. Table 4 presents the results of treatment of this material by the alternative variance method. From the significance value (p) it follows that the probability of appearance of reticulopenia in the test animals in the third month of the experiments was above 99 per cent and in the sixth,

99 per cent. From the material presented it follows that single intratracheal administration of thorium dioxide in an amount up to 400 mg/kg does not produce such sharp depression in erythropoiesis as to lead to development of anaemia in the animals. However, a clear symptom of disturbance in erythropoiesis was change in the number of reticulocytes in the peripheral blood in some test groups. It should be noted that these changes were directly related to the amount of thorium dioxide administered. Thus, in

TABLE 4. *Number of Animals in Fifth and Control Groups with Reticulopenia at Various Times after Administration of* ThO_2

Time after start of experiment in months	% of animals with reticulopenia			
	Controls	Fifth group	t	p
$1\frac{1}{2}$	0–12	30–16	1·5	10%
3	0–12	90–10·6	5·6	1%
5	0–12	33–16·6	1·6	10%
6	10–10	60–17·3	2·5	1%

the animals which were given thorium dioxide in an amount of 2 and 20 mg/kg (first and second groups) no disturbances were observed in erythropoiesis as judged by the tests employed by us (erythrocytes, haemoglobin, reticulocytes). In the animals of the third group (200 mg/kg) the variations in reticulocyte count were greater than in the control group with a certain tendency towards reticulocytosis. However, these changes did not reach the significance level.

Administration of 300 mg/kg thorium dioxide (fourth group) produced in the animals substantial changes in the reticulocyte count with considerable deviation, tending to both rise and fall. It appears that this amount of thorium dioxide brings the erythropoietic system into a state of prolonged functional instability.

Administration of the maximum dose of thorium dioxide in our experiments, namely 400 mg/kg (fifth group), produced periodic reticulopenia which indicated some depression of erythropoietic processes. It is significant that unlike the fourth group (300 mg/kg) no tendency to reticulocytosis was seen in these animals and periodic reticulopenia was the leading symptom.

White Blood

The total leucocyte counts changed to differing extents in the animals of the different groups. Thus, the mean values in the controls and also in the first (2 mg/kg ThO_2) and in the second (20 mg/kg ThO_2) test groups varied within physiological limits peculiar to rats; in the control animals there were from $13,400 \pm 1100$ to $13,400 \pm 950$ leucocytes per mm^3 blood; in the animals of the first group from $13,900 \pm 1000$ to $16,300 \pm 2400$ and in the rats of the second group from $10,500 \pm 940$ to $12,400 \pm 650$. Throughout the experiment no significant changes in the number of leucocytes were observed in the control group. Only in the diseased animals (suppurative bronchitis, focal pneumonia) were solitary cases of leucocytes observed when the count increased to 25,000 per mm^3 blood. Leucocytosis in these cases was of a marked neutrophilic character. The absolute number of neutrophils increased to 10,000–16,000 per mm^3 blood (against the norm of 2000–3000 per mm^3). The absolute number of lymphocytes did not significantly differ from normal and the lymphopenia observed was only relative.

In the first and second groups no significant changes in the total white cell count were observed. There were isolated cases of disease the same as in the control groups. In the diseased animals leucocytosis of the neutrophilic type was observed but together with this we recorded single cases of leucocytosis accompanied by sharp absolute lymphocytosis when the count increased to 18,000–19,000 per mm^3 blood and sometimes even higher. In the animals of the third group (200 mg/kg ThO_2) and the fourth (300 mg/kg ThO_2) solitary cases of leucocytosis with increase in the absolute number of lymphocytes were also observed. However, unlike the animals of the first two groups and the controls they showed a temporary fall in the total number of leucocytes as compared with the initial level; in the third group in the seventh month from $12,700 \pm 840$ down to 8000 ± 220 per mm^3 and in the ninth month up to 9300 ± 470; in the animals of the fourth group the fall occurred somewhat earlier, in the fourth month, but was less marked—from $15,700 \pm 850$ down to $12,700 \pm 860$ per mm^3 blood. As can be seen from these figures, the number of leucocytes remained within the normal lower limits.

Granulocytes

No significant changes in the absolute number of neutrophils were seen throughout the experiment in any of the test groups. In the same way as in the control group, the number of neutrophils was on average from 2500 to 3500 per mm^3 blood except for the cases of neutrophilic leucocytosis noted above. In all the test animals various morphological changes in the cells of the neutrophil series were observed.

The changes in the nuclear structure of the segmented and rod nuclear neutrophils observed in the blood of the control animals and also the animals of the test groups before administration of thorium dioxide were very slight. Thus, only in some animals was fragmentosis of the nucleus observed in 0·3 per cent of the neutrophils. The fragments had the appearance of projecting thorns or, if the disruption was greater, they were joined to the nucleus only by a thin crosspiece. In addition, in normal conditions, usually 1–2 per cent disintegrating neutrophils were encountered.

In the test animals of all groups the number of neutrophils with fragmentosis of the nucleus periodically increased up to 1–1·8 per cent in all animals of some groups. In other groups this increase was observed in most animals (7 or 8 out of 10 animals). The number of disintegrating neutrophils was approximately the same as in the controls.

In the rats treated with thorium dioxide, neutrophils with chromatinolysis of the nucleus were also observed, absent, as a rule, in the control animals. The nucleus lost its typical chromatin structure and was stained homogeneously. The number of such neutrophils periodically reached the range of 0·9—2·7 per cent. The appearance of fragmentosis and chromatinolysis of the nuclei of the neutrophils was not found to depend on the amount of thorium dioxide and the exposure times.

In the test animals hypersegmented neutrophils also appeared (with a number of segments above seven). The size of these cells in most cases was not greater than the usual neutrophils but in single cases giant forms were encountered. The number of hypersegmented forms was not strictly related to the dose of thorium dioxide. The time of appearance in the blood of the hypersegmented forms of neutrophils was rather indefinite and in all groups we observed two maximum rises. Apparently, hypersegmentosis usually develops after 6 months' exposure.

Thus, despite the fact that there were no significant deviations from normal in the absolute numbers of neutrophils in the test animals, we observed a number of qualitative changes of both a degenerative-destructive character (chromatinolysis) and changes possibly associated with disturbed maturation of the neutrophils (hypersegmentosis, fragmentosis).

The number of other granulocytes, eosinophils and basophils, found in the test groups did not significantly differ from their number in the control group.

Lymphocytes

The absolute numbers of lymphocytes expressed as the number per mm^3 blood, in the test groups before administration of thorium dioxide were as follows: in the first group 8700 ± 530, in the second 7300 ± 520, in the third 8500 ± 850, in the fourth $11,600 \pm 840$, in the fifth 9100 ± 670 and in the control group 8800±970. The course of changes in the absolute number of lymphocytes in the test animals after administration of thorium dioxide and also in the control animals is indicated in Fig. 2. In Table 5 the same data is given as a percentage of the initial number of lymphocytes.

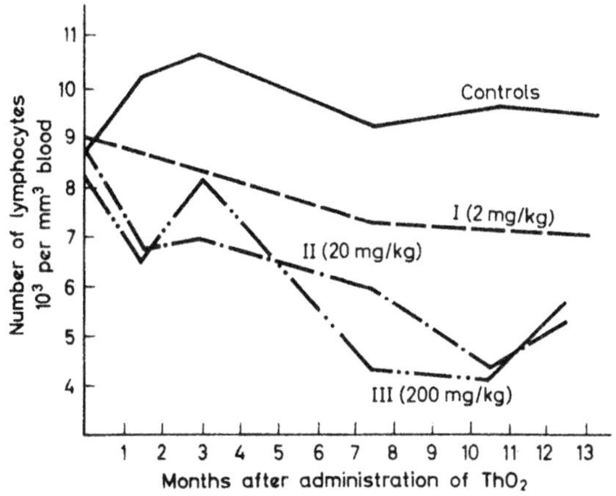

FIG. 2. Change in absolute number of lymphocytes after a single intratracheal administration of thorium dioxide

In the animals of the control group the absolute number of lymphocytes changed throughout the experiment very little. On administration to the test animals of 2 and 20 mg/kg thorium dioxide (first and second groups) no significant deviations were found in the absolute numbers of lymphocytes. As stated above, isolated cases of absolute lymphocytosis were observed (with leucocytosis or a normal number of leucocytes) and after 9–13 months of the experiment 4–5 rats of the group developed absolute lymphopenia with lymphocyte count below 5000 per mm³ blood. However, calculation of the significance coefficient did not confirm the significance of these deviations as compared with the control group.

In the animals given 200 mg/kg thorium dioxide (third group) solitary cases of absolute lymphocytosis were also observed. However, in the great majority of rats 7–8 months after the start of the experiment marked absolute lymphopenia appeared. The minimum number of lymphocytes was in this period 4300±470 per mm³ blood, which corresponds to 51 per cent of the initial value (Fig. 3, Tables 5 and 6). From the 13th month the number of lymphocytes began to return to normal.

In the animals of the fourth group which each received 300 mg/kg thorium dioxide the fall in the lymphocytes began earlier than in the third group. After three months the number of lymphocytes was 68±10·4 per cent of the initial level and after 10 months 57·4±4·4 per cent. There was a relation between the maximum fall in the absolute number of lymphocytes

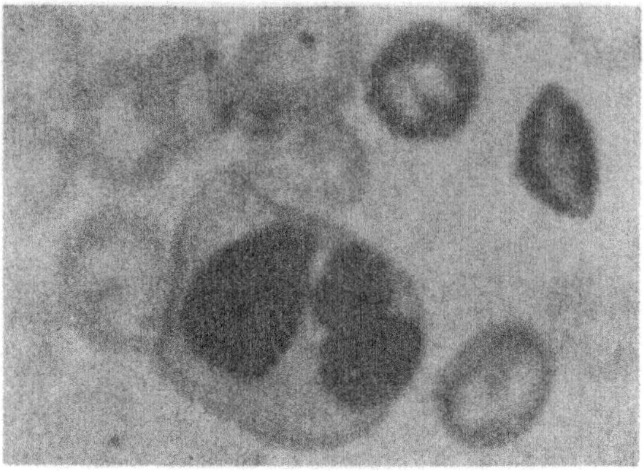

FIG. 3. Trinucleated lymphocyte in peripheral blood of rat No. 103 found in the twelfth month after administration (90×30)

and their initial number: the extent of decrease in the absolute number of lymphocytes in the third to fifth groups which received 200, 300 and 400 mg/kg thorium dioxide was approximately the same and reached 54–57 per cent of the initial level. However, in the animals of the third group which before the experiment had 8500 ± 810 lymphocytes per mm^3 blood, considerable lymphopenia ensued while in the fourth group which had an initial number of lymphocytes 1·5 times higher, lymphopenia was observed only in individual animals. On average the number of lymphocytes in the tenth month for the fourth group was 6800 ± 880 per mm^3 blood.

After administration of thorium dioxide together with quantitative changes certain morphological changes were observed in the lymphocytes. Thus, in all the test groups and usually after 5–9 months of the experiment, vacuolization of the lymphocyte cells was observed mostly affecting the protoplasm and less often the nucleus. Their number on average in the groups was from 0·7 to 1·4 per cent irrespective of the amount of thorium dioxide. Sometimes, such cells were also encountered in the controls but considerably fewer. In addition, at late stages after administration of thorium dioxide (usually after 10–12 months) we observed in the blood of the majority of test animals binucleated lymphocytes (0·8–1·4 per cent on average). The formation of these cells was usually connected with amitotic division (Fig. 3).

There was no significant increase in the number of disintegrating lymphocytes as compared with the controls. However, some increases were observed in some animals of the third to fifth groups in the second–third month of the experiment.

Thus, a significant decrease in the number of lymphocytes in the peripheral blood after intratracheal administration of thorium dioxide to the

TABLE 5. *Change in the Absolute Number of Lymphocytes (as Percentage of the Initial Value) during Chronic Experiments*

Time after start of experiment (in months)	Group											
	First (2 mg/kg ThO_2)		Second (20 mg/kg ThO_2)		Third (200 mg/kg ThO_2)		Fourth (300 mg/kg ThO_2)		Fifth (400 mg/kg ThO_2)		Controls	
	M±m	±σ	M±m	±σ	M±m	±σ	M±m	±σ	M±m	±σ	M±m	±σ
1½	95·3±9·1	28·6	89±4·6	13·3	89·7±12·4	38·6	89·5±12·4	24·8	77·3±8·5	20·5	89·4±12·0	31·4
3	90·2±10	24·0	115·0±9·4	28·2	118·0±11·6	35·9	68·0±10·4	20·9	75·7±8·2	19·8	106·5±14·6	38·0
5	123±9·6	21·2	98·5±8·8	22·0	107·0±8·0	25·0	67·7±5·9	11·8	62·2±5·7	12·5	99·7±10·6	27·5
6	98·5±10·0	26·3	100±10·3	25·5	80·4±11·1	34·3	62·4±13	28·7	71·6±7·9	17·5	96·5±6·8	17·5
8	80·5±5·5	14·3	83·4±9·1	23·7	59·8±6·1	19·4	68·0±8·3	18·2	54·2±11·8	23·7	93·8±4·7	9·6
10	78·2±2·9	7·6	76·0±9·5	24·6	57·1±2	9·0	57·4±4·4	9·8	68·0±8·1	17·9	92·6±9·1	21·8
13	78·4±7·2	17·6	99·2±14·3	28·6	79·2±11·4	25·0	83·6±0·5	10·0	—	—	—	—

TABLE 6. *Change in the Absolute Number of Lymphocytes in Blood of the Animals of the Third Group during Chronic Experiment (per mm³)*

	Before administration of thorium dioxide	Time after administration of thorium dioxide in months							
		1½	3	5	6	7	8	10	13
M±m	8500±850	7500±1300	9400±600	8400±670	6500±890	4800±510	4300±470	6100±350	6600±870
σ±mσ	2700±600	4100± 910	1900±420	2030±480	2820±630	1620±360	1140±400	2980±940	2080±600

rats in our experiments was observed for doses of 200 mg/kg (third group) and higher doses. However, the lymphoid tissue also reacted to smaller amounts of thorium dioxide as indicated by the appearance of morphologically changed lymphocytes at doses of 2 and 20 mg/kg. But we did not observe any intensification of the qualitative changes in the lymphocytes with increase in the dose. The qualitative changes in the cells were approximately the same in the animals of all the test groups. The times of their appearance in most of the animals of the third group were fairly late and corresponded to the start of restoration of the number of lymphocytes. The appearance of binucleated lymphocytes was associated with the onset in this period of increased activity of the lymphoid tissue. Some disturbances in lymphopoiesis in turn might have produced degenerative processes and vacuolization of the lymphoid cells.

Thrombocytes

The number of platelets before the start of the experiment in all animals was fairly high within the limits 500,000–800,000 per mm^3 blood. The time course of the change in the number of thrombocytes during the experiment is indicated in Fig. 4 where the initial number is taken as 100 per cent.

The changes in the platelet count in the animals after administration of 2, 20 and 300 mg/kg thorium dioxide did not significantly differ from the variations in the control group. On administration of 200 mg/kg thorium dioxide a temporary but significant increase in the number was observed.

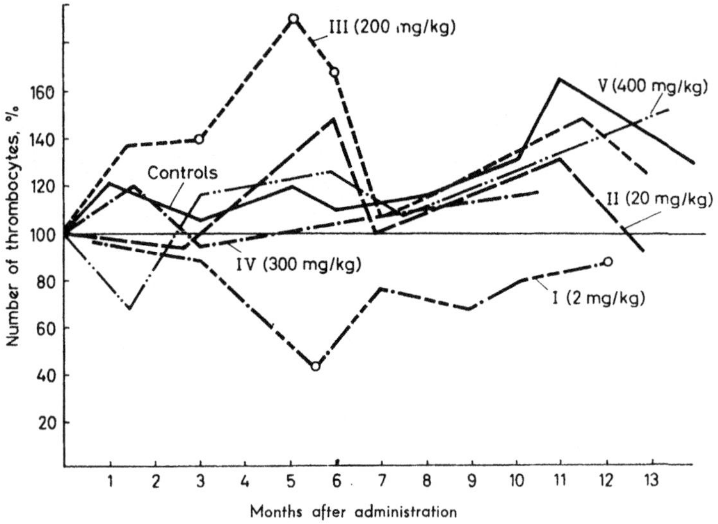

FIG. 4. Change in thrombocyte count (as % of initial value) after single intratracheal administration of thorium dioxide.

In the animals given 400 mg/kg, a persistent fall in the number of blood platelets was observed approximately at the same time. However, this fall may be regarded only as relative since because of the high number of thrombocytes before the experiment (800,000 per mm^3) even with maximum fall in the fifth month their number remained within normal limits (400,000 per mm^3 blood).

TABLE 7. *Change in the Absolute Number of Thrombocytes in Blood of the Animals of the Third and Control Groups (per mm^3)*

Groups	Before experiment	Time in months after administration of 200 mg/kg				
		$1^1/_2$	3	5–6	8	10–11
Test animals of third group	$M \pm m$ 716,000 ±61·000	980,000 ±95,000	1,094,000 ±105,000	1,187,000 ±119,000	734,000 ±61,000	834,000 ±68,000
	$\sigma \pm m\sigma$ 182,000 ±43,000	285,000 ±68,000	315,000 ±75,000	262,000 ±82,000	196,000 ±45,000	178,000 ±48,000
		Months of experiment				
Control animals	$M \pm m$ 577,000 ±46,000	570,000 ±65,000	489,000 ±31,000	620,000 ±72,000	546,000 ±61,000	582,000 ±59,000
	$\sigma \pm m\sigma$ 148,000 ±33,000	170,000 ±46,000	98,000 ±22,000	232,000 ±51,000	182,000 ±43,000	177,000 ±42,000

Table 7 indicates changes in the absolute number of thrombocytes in the third and control groups. The table shows genuine thrombocytosis, indicated by an increase in the number of bood platelets relative to the initial level and that their number increased even above 1 million per mm^3 blood from 3 to 6 months after administration. A further interesting point is that the value of the root mean square deviation (σ) corresponding to the third month rose significantly ($t = 2{\cdot}7$) in the animals of the third group as compared with the controls and again fell by the fifth to sixth month. Consequently change in the number of thrombocytes was accompanied by considerable variation in this index in the same way as was true of the lymphocytes and reticulocytes.

Summary

Summing up the experimental study of the effect of thorium dioxide on certain aspects of haemopoiesis, we may note the following changes in the peripheral blood appearing during 10 to 11 months after intratracheal administration of various amounts of thorium dioxide.

1. Intratracheal administration of thorium dioxide in amounts from 300 to 400 mg/kg body weight produced in the rats a disturbance in erythropoiesis manifest in change in the number of reticulocytes. Thus, a dose of 300 mg/kg ThO_2 produced a state of functional instability expressed in fluctuations in the reticulocyte count wider than in the control animals. Administration of 400 mg/kg caused some depression of erythropoiesis in the form of periodic reticulopenia.

2. Changes in lymphopoiesis were indicated by the relative fall in the absolute numbers of lymphocytes observed even after administration of only 200 mg/kg ThO_2 and also by the appearance of morphologically changed lymphocytes.

3. No quantitative changes in the number of neutrophils were observed. However, the various morphological changes in the nuclei of the neutrophils indicated some disturbance in granulocytopoiesis.

4. The effect of thorium dioxide on thrombocytopoiesis is indicated by the increase, relative to the initial value, in the number of blood platelets after administration of 200 mg/kg thorium dioxide.

5. One of the early reactions of the body to administration of thorium dioxide was instability of haemopoiesis, expressed in considerable variation in the number of reticulocytes, thrombocytes and lymphocytes.

References

BACKER O. G., Peripheral Blood Changes following Internal Contamination with Radioactive Material (Colloidal Thorium Dioxide). *Progress in Radiobiology.* Oliver & Boyd (1956).

BARANSKI S. and BARKOWA O., Sklad Morfologiezni krwi obwodowej i szpico bialych szcurow. *Folia Morphologica* **7,** 2, 109–124 (1956).

DUANE G. W., Aplastic Anaemia Fourteen Years following Administration of Thorotrast. *Amer. J. Med.* **23,** 499–501 (1957).

GEBAUER A. and HEINECKER R., Jatrogene und gewerbliche Radium und Thoriumschaden. *Strahlentherapie*, **98,** 4, 558–569 (1955).

GOTTLIEB R., Effect of Colloidal Thorium on Blood Picture. *Canad. Med. Ass. J.* **28,** 496–497 (1933).

GREBE S. F., Beitrag zur Frage der Thorotrastspätschädigung. Eine myeloische Leukämie nach diagnostischer Thorotrastapplikation. *Strahlentherapie*, **94,** 2, 311–319 (1954).

GROTE W. and PAMPUS F., Beitrage zur Thorotrastschädigung nach Arteriographie der Hirnegfasse. *Arch. klin. Chir.* **281,** 109–119 (1955).

HIERONYMI G. and SANDKÜHLER S., Bone Marrow Insufficiency 11 Years after Use of Thorotrast. *Dtsch. Arch. klin. Med.* **200,** 561–582 (1953).

LAMBIN P. and GERARD M. J., La thrombopenie causée par le dioxyde de thorium colloidal. *Sang*, **6,** 804–808 (1932).

LOONEY W. B., An Investigation of the Late Clinical Findings following Thorotrast (Thorium Dioxide) Administration. *Amer. J. Roentgenol.* **83,** 1, 163–185 (1960).

MAINX F., Radioactive Leuchtfarben in der Uhrenindustrie. *Zbl. Arbeitsened.* **7,** 4, 88–89 (1957).

MOESCHLIN S., MARTI H. R. and GERMANN W., Fatal Panmyelopathy due to Thorotrast. *Schweiz. med. Wschr.* **83,** 1061–1064 (1953).

MONTANARI-REGGIANI M., Contribute sperimentale alla conoscenza delle alterazioni indotte dal nitrato di torie nell organisme animale. *Arch. Ital. Sci. Farmacol.* **2,** 245–263 (1933).

NETOUŠEK M., BORES J. and DVORAK K., Chronic Myelosis following the Use of Thorotrast. *Blood*, **12,** 291 (1957).

SAKHAROV P. P., *Laboratory Animals* (*Laboratory zhivotnye*). Moscow-Leningrad (1952).

SPIER J., CLUFF L. E. and URRY W. D., Aplastic Anaemia following Administration of Thorotrast. *J. Lab. Clin. Med.* **32,** 147–154 (1947).

TARASENKO N. YU., Problem of the Toxicity of Thorium (K voprosu o toksichnosti toriya). *Gig. trud. i profzabolevan.* **6,** 21–27 (1960).

THOMAS S. F., HENRY G. W. and KAPLAN H. S., Hepatolienography; Past, Present and Future. *Radiology*, **57,** 669 (1951).

VIKTOROV K. R., Quoted by NIKITIN V. N., *Atlas of Blood Cells of Farm and Laboratory Animals* (*Atlas kletok krovi selskokhozyaistvennykh i laboratornykh zhivotnykh).* Moscow (1956).

WEIL E. and MENEFRIER, *Sang*, 3, 221–228 (1937).

THE EFFECT OF THORIUM DIOXIDE ON ARTERIAL PRESSURE AND THRESHOLD OF STIMULATION OF THE NERVE-MUSCLE APPARATUS IN RATS

YAN SYAO-SHAN

IN THE literature there is very little information on the nature of the effect of thorium compounds on the cardiovascular system. Watanabe (1957) showed that intravenous injection of 2–3 mg/kg body weight of a solution of thorium chloride into rabbits produces a moderate fall in blood pressure. On injection of the same solution in a dose of 5 mg/kg a transient fall in blood pressure was more obvious and with increase in the dose to 10 mg/kg the fall in blood pressure was considerable. Sometimes the sharp drop in blood pressure was the cause of death of the animal.

Timokhin (1958) reported on 19 cases of hypotension among 25 workers examined by him and who for a long time had been engaged in the production of a catalyst containing thorium, cobalt and magnesium. He observed in these workers symptoms of disturbance in autonomic innervation, change in the skin-vascular reactions, etc. Although he emphasized the danger of exposure of workers to thorium aerosols, it should not be forgotten that as well as thorium the catalyst contained cobalt and magnesium and, therefore, in analysis of the results it is necessary to make an experimental study of the effect of each component on the animal body.

Experiments carried out on frogs, rabbits and cats (Watanabe, 1957) and also on dogs (Frolova, 1960) showed the damaging effect of thorium on the circulatory system. Thus, for example, in experiments with perfusion of the isolated cat heart with Ringer's solution containing thorium chloride in a dose of 0·01 mg Watanabe (1957) observed a moderate fall in the amplitude of contraction of the heart. With increase in the dose of thorium to 0·1 mg, the amplitude of ventricular contraction fell while for the atrium it increased. When thorium chloride was added to Ringer's solution in an amount of 1 mg the amplitude of both fell with disturbance in the conductivity of excitation in the heart. The author also obtained similar results in frog experiments. From these experimental results Watanabe concluded that definite amounts of thorium exert a negative chronotropic and dromotropic effect on the isolated heart of both cold and warm-blooded animals.

Frolova (1960) carried out an experiment on dogs which were given different doses of thorium fluoride by inhalation in order to study the ECG in these animals. The adrenalin load revealed signs of toxic effect of thorium on the dog heart. The animals showed extrasystole, total and partial AV block, temporary paroxysmal tachycardia, auricular fibrillation and heterotropic foci of excitation. In a number of dogs the increase in the T-wave in the period of vagal inhibition was more marked than normal. Thus, the changes revealed by the functional adrenalin load point to disturbances in the excitability, conductivity and automatism of the heart produced by the thorium fluoride.

Analysing these few published findings it may be said that they refer only to certain thorium compounds. We have no information on the effect of thorium oxide on the cardiovascular system. Yet ThO_2, like other thorium compounds, may change the activity of this system and in particular, influence arterial pressure. Accordingly, we set out to study the effect on the arterial pressure in rats of thorium dioxide by intratracheal and intraperitoneal administration.

Effect of Thorium Dioxide on Arterial Pressure in Rats

The arterial systolic pressure was measured in eight groups of 10 rats each in a chronic experiment for 18 months after administration of thorium dioxide via the trachea (1st–5th) and intraperitoneally (6th and 7th). The 8th group was the control.

A number of workers (Byrom and Wilson, 1938; Williams, Harrison and Grollman, 1939; Chernov, 1947; Kogan, 1950) have proposed various modifications of the bloodless method for experimental determination of arterial pressure. We used this method as modified by Kogan with certain variations. Its advantages are simplicity and the possibility of measuring the blood pressure without anaesthesia in a chronic experiment, which comes closer to physiological conditions.

The arterial pressure was determined in 57 normal rats for two weeks before administration of thorium dioxide to establish the norm. In all, we made 149 measurements at intervals from 1 to 13 days. The results show that in 71 per cent of all the measurements the value of arterial pressure was within the limits of 91–110 mm Hg, which is in agreement with the results obtained by a number of workers who have used this method. For example, the arterial pressure reading in rats according to Williams *et al.* (1939) varies from 100 to 125 mm Hg, according to Chernov (1947) from 80 to 110 mm, according to Kogan (1950) from 100 to 130 mm and

Zakharov (1960) from 100 to 130 mm Hg. A certain disparity in the findings obtained by different workers is possibly to be explained by the different sensitivity of the plethysmographs used. In our investigations we started from the values obtained by us for the arterial pressure of the rat tail in normal conditions, 91–110 mm Hg.

The results obtained in the experimental rats during 18 months' observation are given in Table 1.

TABLE 1. *Course of Change in Arterial Systolic Pressure in Rats in millimetres Mercury Column (Mean data for rats after intratracheal (Groups 1–5) and intraperitoneal (Group 6) administration of* ThO_2*)*

Time after administration in months	Groups						
	I	II	III	IV	V	VI[a]	VIII
	2 mg/kg	20 mg/kg	200 mg/kg	300 mg/kg	400 mg/kg	1000 mg/kg	Control 1 ml saline per rat
Before administration	91·5	92·2	99	94·3	96	94·4	96
$1^1/_2$	94	90	96	97·7	95·5	95·9	90
3	94·8	98	90	95·3	103·6	110·1	93
4	92	—	94	99·4	—	97·2	91
5	95	92	93	90·2	90·7	98·6	90
6	—	93	98	91·5	73·9 ±2·16	99·6 ±5·8	—
7	93·4 ±1·38	99	99·2	65·8±0·8	64·3±5·4	73·7±5·1	94±0·95
8	96·2	96·7	97·4	70	72·4	68·4	98·2
9	96·1	98	91·1	68·3	62	61·7	99
10	—	—	97·5	65·3	56	—	89·7
11	79·5	83·7	87·0	71	—	—	85·8
12	55·3±5·7	69·2±2·7	46·7±4·3	69±3·8	64·5±2·3	52·0±6·0	89·6±2·4
13	56·1	68	57·5	57·8	60·8	52·7	81·5
14	53·5	59·3	58	58	—	55	80·3
15	57·6	63·2	60·6	56·5	54·8	54·6	84·2
16	52·3	56·5	60·2	—	—	—	86·6
17	63·3	54·2	60·2	—	—	55·8	80·2
18	50·0	48	57·5	54	43·7	—	77

[a] In view of the uniformity of findings for groups VI and VII, the findings for group VII are not given.

As the table shows, the arterial pressure in the control (8th) group was quite constant throughout the observation period. Only at certain periods (13 months after the start of the experiment) was there some deviation from the initial level (fall to 80 mm Hg).

A different picture was observed in rats treated with thorium dioxide.

As Fig. 1 shows, in those receiving ThO_2 in doses of 200 mg/kg and less, the arterial pressure for a long time (up to 11 months) varied within normal limits. Twelve months after administration it began to show a considerable and steady fall reaching 55–60 mm Hg and in individual rats even 40 mm Hg. The difference in arterial pressure in the control and test animals on statistical treatment of the results was significant. However, no distinct relation could be seen between the fall in arterial pressure and dose. Subsequently, hypotension was noted throughout the period of investigation without any tendency to return to normal.

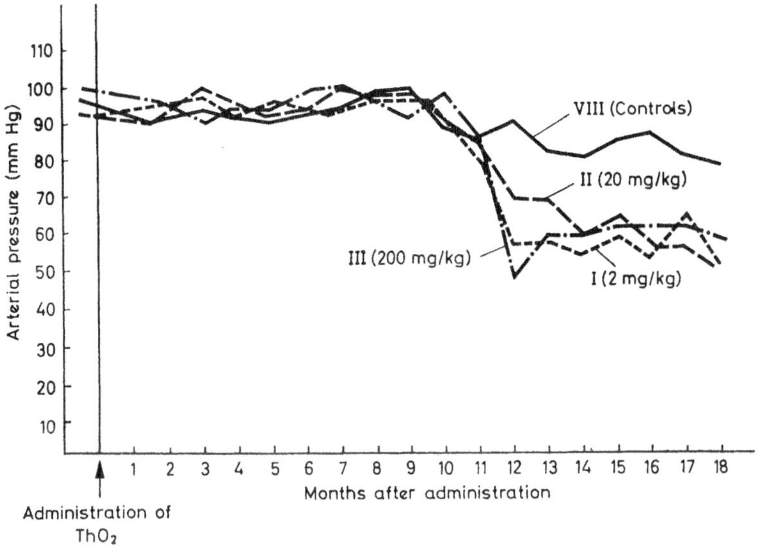

FIG. 1. Course of changes in arterial pressure in rats after single intratracheal administration of thorium dioxide (groups I, II, III and VIII)

The results of investigation of arterial pressure in rats receiving thorium oxide in large doses and by different routes of administration are depicted in Fig. 2 where it will be seen that the course of arterial pressure in the rats given thorium oxide in doses of 300, 400 and 1000 mg/kg differed little from that for lower doses. The difference was most apparent for the onset of hypotension. Thus, in the 4th and 6th groups it appeared after 6–7 months' exposure, i.e. considerably earlier than in the 1st–3rd groups where the fall in blood pressure began only after 11–12 months. Return to normal was not observed in any test animals throughout 18 months' observation.

Comparing the course of change in blood pressure in the rats of the 4th–6th groups it may be seen that on intraperitoneal injection of thorium oxide (1000 mg/kg) despite the high dose of substance introduced, the

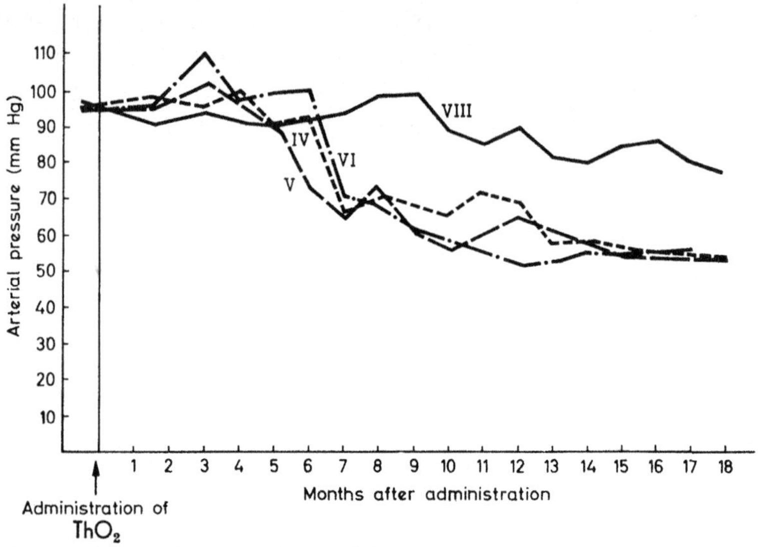

FIG. 2. Course of changes in arterial pressure in rats after single intratracheal injection of thorium dioxide (groups IV, V, VI, VIII)

arterial pressure began to fall somewhat later than in the animals receiving an amount of 400 mg/kg intratracheally.

Analysis of the results allows us to relate the fall in arterial pressure observed in the rats to the effect of thorium dioxide. The basis for this is provided by our own experimental findings showing the relative stability of blood pressure in the controls during 18 months and considerable fall in animals receiving intratracheal and intraperitoneal injection of thorium dioxide. Indirect proof of the phenomenon observed by us is afforded by published findings. Thus, Timokhin (1958) found that the blood pressure of workers in contact with thorium at work begins to fall with disturbance in autonomic regulation. This is also indicated by the experimental observations of Watanabe (1957). Thus, as a result of the prolonged action of thorium dioxide given intratracheally and intraperitoneally there is irreversible fall in arterial pressure in rats.

Effect of Thorium Dioxide on the Stimulation Threshold of the Nerve-muscle Apparatus of Animals

In the literature available we have found no information on the effect of thorium on the central nervous system and therefore decided to determine the stimulation thresholds of the nerve-muscle apparatus in dynamic conditions in rats taking it as a pointer to the state of the central nervous system.

The principle of the method employed by us consists in determination of the minimum voltage of electric current which in a single exposure may produce in rats contraction of the muscle-flexors of the toes of the hind limbs. The investigation was carried out by means of a combined electrometronome.

The electrometronome consists of three parts: (1) a rectifying device supplying the anode and filament circuits; (2) a sound frequency oscillatory generator constructed from a 6N8S double triode and a 6N8S valve post-amplifier; (3) the output part which makes it possible to obtain signals both in the form of sound vibrations and as electric pulses corresponding to them. The experimenter can regulate at will the frequency of the sound vibrations. Copper electrodes are attached to the instrument which are covered with gauze and constantly wetted with physiological saline. For determining the threshold of stimulation of the nerve-muscle apparatus of rats the experimenter attaches the hind limbs of the rats to the electrodes. The response to stimulation is recorded from the twitch of the muscle-flexors of the toes. With minimum frequency of electric pulses (30 per min) by changing the resistance we determined the minimal voltage capable of eliciting a twitch of the muscles of the toes. To avoid a summation effect each subsequent stimulation was applied only after 0·5 min.

The stimulation threshold was determined in the same groups of rats in which blood pressure had been investigated. The determinations were made during 18 months after intratracheal and intraperitoneal administration of thorium oxide, at first twice a month and every month after three months.

Before administration of thorium oxide we determined in 140 rats the stimulation threshold of the nerve-muscle apparatus of the hind paws. In all, 400 measurements were made. It was established that the stimulation threshold using this apparatus in white rats in normal conditions was expressed by a voltage of $13{\cdot}83 \pm 1{\cdot}55$ relative units of the instrument.

The results obtained in the test rats during 18 months are presented in Table 2.

As can be seen from the table, in the animals of all groups during the 18 months' observation period the threshold of stimulation of the nerve-muscle apparatus of the paw was fairly constant, i.e. varied within narrow limits. These results suggest absence of appreciable changes in the central nervous system in rats treated with thorium dioxide.

Taking into account the considerable changes in blood pressure in the test rats it may be assumed that the autonomic sections of the central nervous system regulating the vascular system are affected earlier and to a greater degree.

TABLE 2. *Course of Changes in Stimulation Threshold of Nerve-muscle Apparatus of White Rats after Administration of* ThO_2 *(in relative units of voltage averaged for 10 rats)*

Time of measurement after administration in months	Groups						
	I	II	III	IV	V	VI	VIII
	Dose of ThO_2 in mg/kg						
	2	20	200	300	400	1000	Controls
Before administration	13·0	13·7	12·6	14·6	14·2	15·2	13·3
½	12·9	12·5	12·6	—	14·3	—	—
1	13·1	13·2	12·9	14·7	14·6	14·9	12·8
2	12·9	13·6	13·1	14·2	13·5	14·0	12·5
3	13·7	13·9	13·5	15·1	14·3	14·1	12·9
4	14·0	14·0	13·1	14·7	14·8	14·4	13·9
5	12·7	13·5	14·0	14·6	14·0	—	—
6	12·8	14·6	13·9	14·5	14·3	—	13·7
7	14·3	14·3	13·6	13·2	—	13·9	13·7
8	13·8	—	14·2	—	14·5	—	13·8
9	—	13·8	13·9	—	—	14·0	13·8
10	13·1	—	14·7	14·0	14·0	14·5	13·6
11	—	13·6	14·5	15·6	14·6	14·4	—
12	14·3	13·8	—	13·8	—	14·0	—
13	14·0	—	14·4	14·1	15·0	—	—
14	13·6	14·0	13·7	15·1	—	14·4	14·6
15	13·7	14·4	14·0	15·4	—	—	15·2
16	14·4	14·8	14·0	—	—	—	15·2
17	15·8	14·6	15·4	—	—	—	14·8
18	16·0	15·4	16·2	—	—	—	15·0

Summary

1. Intratracheal and intraperitoneal injection of thorium dioxide in doses of 2, 20, 200, 300, 400 and 1000 mg/kg produce a sharp and persistent fall in arterial pressure in rats.

2. The stimulation threshold of the muscle-nerve apparatus of the hind paws in rats treated with thorium dioxide showed no significant changes during 18 months' observation.

References

BYROM T. W. and WILSON C., A Plethysmographic Method for Measuring Systolic Blood Pressure in the Intact Rat. *J. Physiol.* **93,** 3, 301–304 (1938).

CHERNOV V. M., O metodakh nekrovavogo opredeleniya krovyanogo davleniya u melkikh laboratornykh zhivotnykh v khronicheskikh opytakh (Methods of Bloodless

Determination of Blood Pressure in Small Laboratory Animals in Chronic Experiments). *Farmakologiya i toksikologiya*, **X**, 2, 39–44 (1947).

FROLOVA I. A., Respredeleniye in vyvedeniye toriya u krys pri intratrakheal'nom vvedenii ego nerastvorimoi soli (Distribution and Elimination of Thorium in Rats on Intratracheal Administration of its Insoluble Salts). *Collection of Abstracts on Radiation Medicine for 1957*, Vol. 1, pp. 131–132. Medgiz (1959).

FROLOVA I. A., Izmeneniya elektrokardiogrammy u sobak, satravlennykh toriyem (Changes in the ECG in Dogs Burdened with Thorium). *Meditsineskaya radiologiya*, **5**, 10, 79 (1960).

KOGAN A. KH., Znachenie beremennosti v razvitii ekspereimntal'noi pochechnoi gipertonii (The Importance of Pregnancy in the Development of Experimental Renal Hypertension). Thesis, Moscow (1950).

TIMOKHIN D. I., Komplekenoye izucheniye uslovii truda i sostoyaniya zdorov'ya rabochykh proizvodstva katalizatora (Comprehensive Study of the Working Conditions and State of Health of Workers in Catalyst Production). *Information Bulletin of theF. F. Erisman Institute*, **16**, 55–62 (1958).

WATANABE S., Pharmacological and Toxicological Studies on Thorium, a Rare Earth Metal. *J. Tokyo Med. College*, **15**, 2, 121–439 (1957).

WILLIAMS J. R., HARRISON T. R. and GROLLMAN A., A Simple Method for Determining The Systolic Blood Presure on the Unanaesthetized Rat. *J. Clin. Invest.* **18**, 3, 373–376 (1939).

ZAKHAROV V. M., Ob izmeneniyakh vyesshei nervnoi deyatel'nosti i arterial'nogo devleniya pri deistvii na organizm malykh doz vnutrennogo oblucheniya natriem-24 (Changes in Higher Nervous Activity and Arterial Pressure on Exposure to Low Dose Internal Irradiation with Sodium-24). Thesis, Moscow (1959).

MORPHOLOGICAL CHANGES IN THE LUNGS AND OTHER ORGANS IN RATS ON INTRATRACHEAL ADMINISTRATION OF THORIUM DIOXIDE

E. S. GAIDOVA and YAN SYAO-SHAN

THE reports published in the literature mainly refer to clinical observations on humans who were injected for diagnostic purposes intravenously with Thorotrast, a preparation of colloidal thorium dioxide, and in part, to experimental investigations on animals.

On intravenous injection, thorium oxide selectively moves towards organs which are rich in reticulo-endothelial elements where it is retained for a long time. Amory (1948), Fonio (1947), Waschulewski (1956) and Brunner (1960) observed development of granulomatous proliferations of the soft tissues appearing at the portals of entry of Thorotrast. In the literature these granulomas produced by thorium have been called thorotrastomas. Mora (1940) and Brody and Cullen (1957) described thorotrastomas in the breast 17 years after mammography using Thorotrast. Thorotrastomas have also been found in the abdominal cavity in the serosa of the lesser pelvis, in the region of the vermiform process, on the surface of the adnexa of the uterus and in the Fallopian tubes after salpingography and intraperitoneal injection of Thorotrast (Vogtlin and Minder, 1952; Brunner *et al.*, 1957).

Rudolphi (1950) observed in one patient cancer of the eyelid 35 years after local injection of Thorotrast. Moeschlin *et al.*, (1953) and Netoušek (1957) described panmyelopathy and chronic myelosis, appearing 23 years after hepatolienography. The literature contains many reports on development of sarcomas of the liver and bile ducts and carcinomas of the liver (McMahon *et al.*, 1947; Grossiard *et al.*, 1956; and Batzenschlager, 1950). According to Bauer (1959) tumours develop at the sites of deposition of thorium and are often combined with fibrous changes in the organ. The latent period of onset of these tumours was on average 12–18 years.

A number of investigators have published communications on the appearance in rats and mice of sarcomas after subcutaneous injections of Thorotrast (Selbie, 1936, 1938; Prussia, 1936; Bogliolo, 1938; Miyumoto,

1939). Roussy *et al.* (1934) were the first to find experimentally that on introducing thorium dioxide into the peritoneal cavity of rats a tumour was produced in these animals. The work of Foulds (1939) is of interest. The author introduced 0·2–0·3 ml Thorotrast into the mammary glands of guinea pigs. On average, 37 months after injection in two of nine animals sarcomas appeared, in one, carcinoma and in another, fibrosarcoma. The first three tumours could be transplanted by the author in 15 passages.

Guimares *et al.*, (1955) observed degenerative and necrotic changes in the hepatic and Kupffer cells and also in the tissue of the spleen. Tumours due to incorporated Thorotrast appear in rats on average after 320 days and in rabbits after 2–3 years (Johnsen, 1954).

The picture of damage to the body from thorium entering via the respiratory tract has received little study.

Tarasenko (1960) showed that on intratracheal administration to rats of an insoluble thorium compound (fluoride) in an amount (calculated for thorium) of 65 mg/kg weight, leucocytosis developed during the first month of treatment. Pathological changes in the internal organs were also noted expressed in degenerative changes with predominant involvement of the lungs, liver and kidneys. The author did not observe tumour development.

The effect on the body of insoluble thorium compounds, especially its dioxide via the respiratory tract has received nothing like sufficient attention, although this route is the most realistic one for workers in contact with thorium in its extraction and use.

The present investigation was carried out on male white rats weighing 250–300 g. The animals were divided into five groups, 20 per group. The test rats (1st–4th groups) were given a single intratracheal administration of a suspension of thorium dioxide in physiological saline in an amount of 2, 20, 200 and 300 mg per kg body weight, or respectively $19{\cdot}2\times10^{-5}$, $19{\cdot}2\times10^{-4}$, $19{\cdot}2\times10^{-3}$ and $29{\cdot}0\times10^{-3}$ μCi per kg weight. These amounts were roughly 0·25, 2·5, 25 and 37 of the maximum permissible concentrations of thorium for single entry into the human lungs (according to Gusev, 1956). The volume of the suspension administered did not exceed 1 ml. In the control group, rats were given intratracheally the same volume of physiological saline.

A morphological study was made of the organs from 52 test and 12 control rats. The animals which died were autopsied immediately, the others killed by decapitation 6, 13, 18 and 21 months after intratracheal administration of thorium oxide. At each stage there were 2–4 animals per group. For the histological investigation, we took tissue fragments from the lungs, bifurcation lymph nodes, liver, spleen, kidneys, intestines, heart muscle and testes and fixed them in 12 per cent neutral formalin. The usual alcohol stages were observed and the material embedded in celloidin. The sections were stained with haematoxylin and eosin by the method of Perles for iron. Some of the sections from the lungs and individual tumours were additionally stained with picrofuchsin to detect collagen structures.

First Group (rats receiving intratracheally 2 mg/kg ThO_2)

Macroscopic investigation of the organs of animals killed 6 months after treatment did not reveal any pathological lesions. In the lungs histological investigation showed focal emphysema, non-uniform filling of the vessels with blood and small (round-cell) lymphoid infiltrates around the bronchi. In some bronchi hypertrophy of the epithelium was noted. No traces of thorium were found in the lungs. In the regional lymph nodes and internal organs pathological lesions were absent. Thirteen months after treatment the rat lungs were found to contain focal indurations of the interalveolar septa, zones of emphysema and peribronchial lymphoid infiltrates. In individual bronchi, chronic catarrhal-desquamative bronchitis could be seen. In the spleen there were single foci of myeloid haemopoiesis. In the other internal organs no pathological changes were found.

After 19–21 months there was considerable decline in nutrition and alopecia. Macroscopically in the lungs in some of the animals small abscesses were visible with a yellowish-white, often crumblike content. In other organs macroscopically no pathological changes were found except in two rats (Nos. 6 and 18).

Histological inspection of the lungs disclosed focal sclerosis and emphysema more marked than in the early stages. In some of the animals focal chronic productive pneumonia was observed with bronchiectasis, purulent bronchitis and around some of the bronchi adenomatous proliferations and foci of necrosis. In the regional lymph nodes there was slight hyperplasia of the reticulo-endothelial elements. Moderately marked sclerotic changes were seen in the other internal organs.

In rat No. 6 in the region of the right femur a solid, fairly immobile tumour was observed fused with the skin. In cross section the tissue of the tumour was alveolar and sharply plethoric. On histological examination the lesions in the lungs and internal organs of this animal were similar to those described above. The tumour tissue consisted of cavernous cavities of different sizes and shape lined with endothelium and filled with adhering erythrocytes separated by thin connective tissue septa with spindle cells among the fibres (Fig. 1). The femoral bone was not damaged.

In rat No. 18 killed while dying, in the region of the right femur there was a solid-elastic mobile tumour fused with the skin and measuring $1{\cdot}5 \times 2{\cdot}5 \times 3$ cm. At autopsy in the lungs against a background of abscessing pneumonia, individual tumour-like nodules could be seen. A tumour

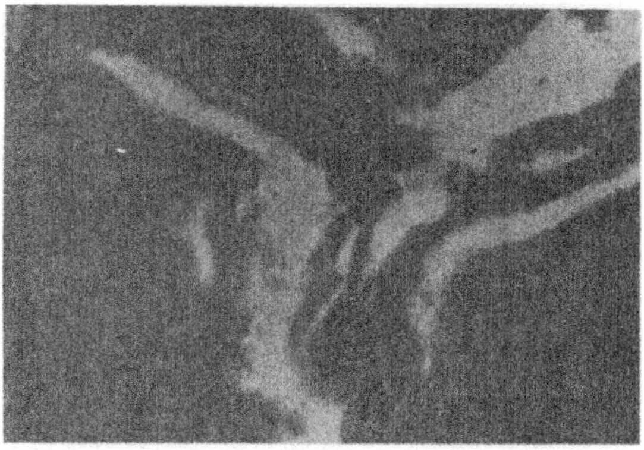

FIG. 1. Photomicrograph of a tumour showing large cavities filled with erythrocytes—cavernous angioma (rat No. 6). Staining with haematoxylin-eosin (×180)

nodule the size of a millet seed was found under the epicardium in the region of the apex of the heart and at the upper pole of the left kidney. An extensive tumour was found retroperitoneally. Histological examination showed that it had the structure of microcellular cancer.

Histological inspection of the lungs revealed focal purulent pneumonia and purulent bronchitis. In some visual fields there were tumourlike proliferations growing through the walls of the bronchi and spreading to the pulmonary tissue consisting of small and medium misshapen epithelial cells often with mitoses arranged in groups among a large number of connective tissue fibres; in individual zones the tumour sharply compressed the bronchi and vessels (Fig. 2). In the regional lymph nodes sharp hyperplasia of the reticuloendothelium was found. In the heart under the epicardium there was a tumourlike nodule consisting of misshapen epithelial cells invading

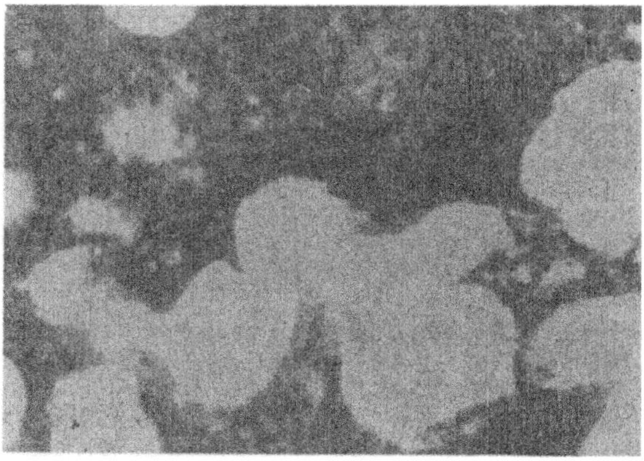

FIG. 2. Photomicrograph of lung. Foci of tumour consisting of small atypical epithelial cells (rat No. 18). Staining with haematoxylin-eosin (×300)

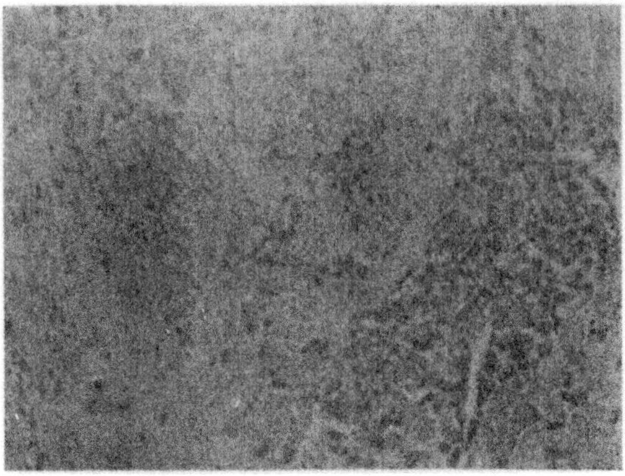

FIG. 3. Photomicrograph. Metastasis of tumour to heart muscle (rat No. 18). Staining with haematoxylin-eosin (×250)

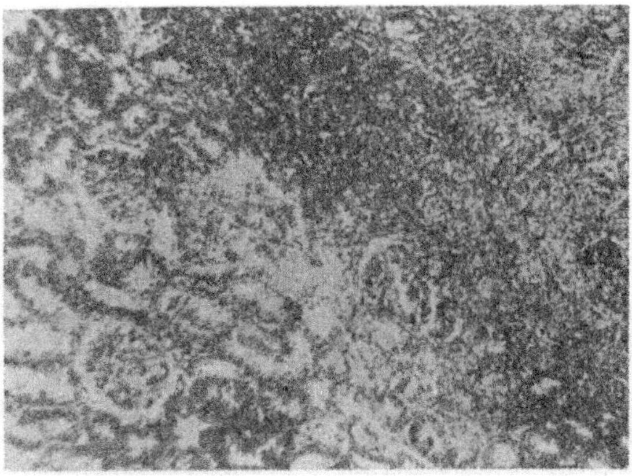

FIG. 4. Photomicrograph of metastasis of lung tumour to kidney tissue (rat No. 16). Staining with haematoxylin-eosin (×180)

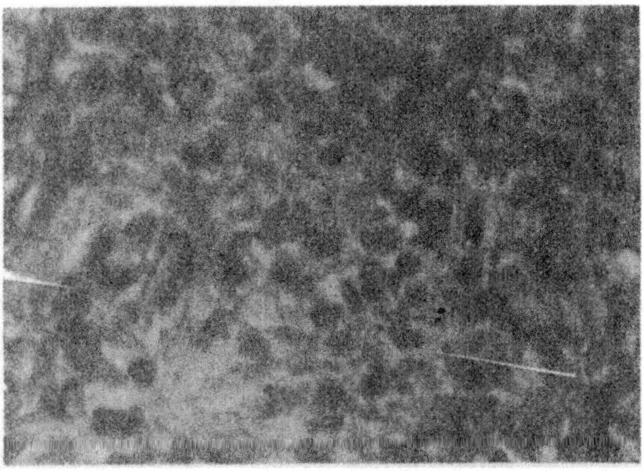

FIG. 5. Photomicrograph of tumour of femoral region consisting of misshapen epithelial cells with numerous mitoses (rat No. 18). Staining with haematoxylin-eosin (×450)

the muscle fibres (Fig. 3). In the kidney there was granular dystrophy and tumour metastasis to the cortical layer (Fig. 4).

The tissue fragments taken from the tumour near the femur and the retroperitoneal tumour consisted of a large number of coarse connective tissue fibres forming in places continuous cicatricial fields among which were honeycombs of misshapen epithelial cells with mitoses (Fig. 5). Apparently, microcellular cancer of the lungs was present with extensive metastases.

Second Group (rats receiving intratracheally 20 mg/kg ThO_2)

In the organs of the animals killed after 6 months of exposure, macroscopic examination indicated no appreciable pathological lesions. Only in the lungs against a background of weakly marked emphysema was it possible to note (chiefly on the posterior surface) small grey nodules which were concentrated in the region of the lung portals.

Microscopic investigation showed the presence in the lungs of weakly marked focal sclerosis and emphysema. Around the small and medium bronchi and in places in the alveolar septa, rare, loose chestnut-brown conglomerations of thorium were seen arranged among the connective tissue fibres with a weak histiocytic reaction at the periphery. There were lymphoid infiltrates around the large bronchi. In the regional lymph nodes and internal organs no appreciable pathological deviations were observed.

After 13 months' exposure the macroscopic and microscopic lesions in the lungs and other organs were very similar to those found after 6 months except in rat No. 21 killed in the agonal state, in which there was a tumour in the left femoral region. Macroscopically, it was possible to see that in the lungs the emphysematous areas alternated with multiple small abscesses with patchy plethora of the internal organs and considerable enlargement of the inguinal and retroperitoneal lymph nodes.

Histological inspection of the tumour of the femoral region gave a diagnosis of spindle cell sarcoma which consisted of chaotically arranged, misshapen spindle cells and fibres with numerous mitoses (Fig. 6).

The inguinal and retroperitoneal lymph nodes were in the form of continuous tumourlike tissue of similar histological structure. In the lungs against a background of purulent pneumonia, bronchiectasis and focal sclerosis it was possible to see extensive regions of metastasis of the tumour with the structure described above.

The spleen was oedematous with hyperplasia of the reticulo-endothelium and foci of myeloid haemopoiesis. In the liver and kidneys there was granular dystrophy.

After 21–22 months' exposure some of the animals died from abscessing

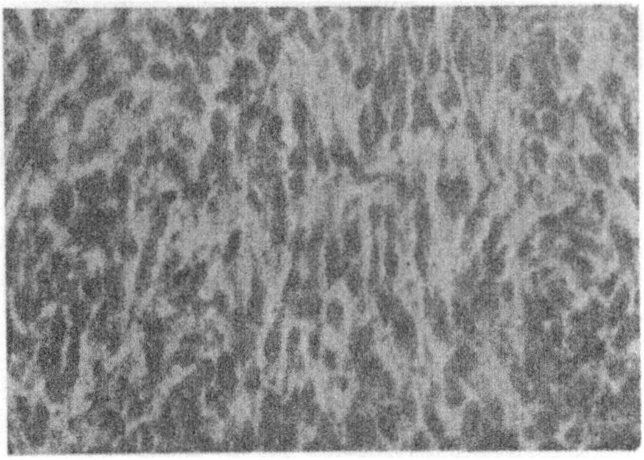

FIG. 6. Photomicrograph of tumour tissue in femoral region. Spindle cell sarcoma (rat No. 21). Staining with haematoxylin-eosin (×450)

pneumonia. In one of the dead rats in the right lung as well as abscesses, a solid tumourlike formation the size of a cherry stone was found. In the killed animals no gross pathological lesions of the organs were seen.

In the killed animals histological examination revealed in the lungs focal sclerosis and emphysema, catarrhal-desquamative bronchitis and moderate hyperplasia of the peribronchial and perivascular lymphoid tissue. Around the individual bronchi and also in the alveolar septa there were small accumulations of the substance administered in the form of chestnut-brown clumps surrounded by hyalinized connective tissue fibres. In the internal organs moderately marked sclerotic and dystrophic lesions were observed. In the lungs of the dead animals we saw chronic purulent bronchitis, perifocal purulent pneumonia, bronchiectasis, adenomatosis, considerable hyperplasia of the peribronchial lymphoid tissue and small accumulations of thorium. In rat No. 38 as well as this against a background of pneumonia there were foci of necrosis and massive areas of sclerosis, consisting of coarse connective tissue fibres among which were honeycombs consisting of atypical flat epithelial cells of the squamous cell cancer type with misshapen nuclei and mitoses.

Third Group (rats receiving 200 mg/kg ThO_2)

Six months after treatment macroscopic investigation of the lungs of these animals pointed against a background of emphysema to small grey nodules arranged chiefly at the portals of the lungs on their posterior surface. In other organs no exceptional changes were seen.

At histological examination we found in the lungs focal emphysema, thickening of the alveolar septa through multiplication of histiocytic elements and sclerosis. The epithelium of the bronchi was succulent and high and considerable hyperplasia of the peribronchial lymphoid tissue could be seen. There were small accumulations of histiocytes around the vessels. Around the bronchi, in the alveolar septa small and large accumulations of thorium were found in the form of coarse amorphous clumps of chest-nut-brown colour; between and around them were thin connective tissue fibres and solitary histiocytes. In the regional lymph nodes moderate hyperplasia of the reticulo-endothelial elements was observed. No severe pathological lesions were found in the internal organs.

After 13 months' exposure macroscopic examination showed in the lungs of some of the animals besides the substance administered small abscesses with some enlargement of the regional lymph nodes and congestive plethora of the internal organs.

Histological examination of the lungs demonstrated focal emphysema, bronchiectasis, catarrhal-purulent bronchitis with a well-marked neutrophilic reaction and peribronchial pneumonia with adenomatosis.

Around some bronchi and in the alveolar septa it was possible to see large and small focal accumulations of thorium between the clumps of which coarse connective tissue fibres in places hyalinized and solitary histiocytes could be seen.

In the regional lymph nodes hyperplasia of the reticulo-endothelial elements was noted and in individual fields it was possible to see extensive conglomerations of thorium in the macrophage or in the form of free clumps in the dilatated vessels. In the spleen there was sharp plethora and foci of myeloid haemopoiesis. Dystrophic changes were found in the liver and kidneys.

After 18–21 months' exposure all the animals were in a poor nutritional state and beginning to lose hair. Macroscopically in all the animals zones of condensation and large abscesses could be seen in the lungs. In addition, in the lungs of rats Nos. 46 and 50 solid tumour-like formations measuring $1{\cdot}5 \times 2{\cdot}5$ cm were found. In rat No. 42 killed in a severe state after 21 months, abscessing pneumonia was found as well as extensive ulcerations of the mucosa of the caecum and considerable enlargement of the right testis, the histological features of which are given below.

Histological examination of the lungs revealed moderate, diffuse sclerosis, emphysema, bronchiectasis, purulent bronchitis, perifocal suppurative desquamative bronchopneumonia, extensive peribronchial conglomerations of lymphoid tissue, solitary plasma cells, small foci of myeloid haemopoiesis and adenomatosis. In the alveolar septa, around the large and medium bronchi there were focal conglomerations of thorium surrounded by coarse connective tissue fibres. In two rats (Nos. 46 and 50) numerous foci of bronchogenic squamous-cell cancer were noticed in places with typical "pearls" formation (Fig. 7). In one rat in the regional lymph node a meta-

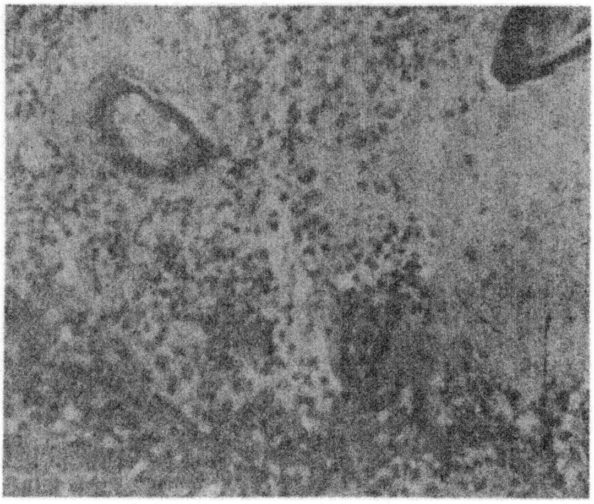

FIG. 7. Photomicrograph of lung tissue. Islets of squamous multilayered epithelium, necroses with central zones of keratinization (rat No. 46). Staining with haematoxylin-eosin (×180)

stasis was found. In the spleens of the animals of this group, oedema was observed. Also in the spleens, among the reticular fibres of the pulp, was a mass of erythrocytes and clumps of chestnut-brown pigment giving a reaction for iron. Small foci of myeloid haemopoiesis were seen.

In the liver, granular dystrophy of the protoplasm of the hepatic cells was observed with small focal necroses. In the kidneys granular dystrophy was seen in the epithelium of the convoluted tubules. There were no marked pathological lesions in the other organs.

In rat No. 42 as well as the above-described lesions in the lungs and organs there was an ulcerative defect of the caecal mucosa with extensive neutrophil infiltration of the submucosa and muscularis. In addition, in the right testis which was considerably enlarged, normal tissue was ab-

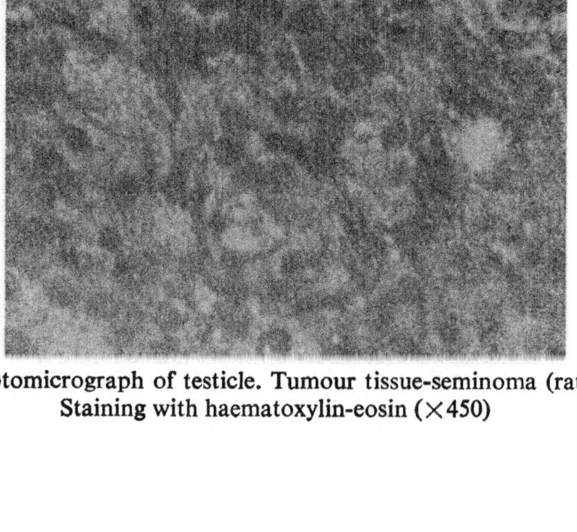

FIG. 8. Photomicrograph of testicle. Tumour tissue-seminoma (rat No. 42). Staining with haematoxylin-eosin (×450)

sent with a few compressed tubules only in one part of the preparation while a seminoma type tumour filled all the other visual fields. The tumour was composed of large cells with frothy protoplasm with bright and eccentric nuclei. Between the cells there were delicate connective tissue fibres. The tissue of the tumour did not penetrate the membranes of the testicle (Fig. 8). The left testis was of normal histological structure.

Fourth Group (rats receiving 300 mg/kg ThO_2)

No animals were killed 6 months after treatment. After 12–13 months' exposure of this group macroscopic inspection of the lungs showed against a background of emphysema small foci of condensation and scattered grey nodules of the administered substance. In other organs no pathological lesions were found. One rat (No. 89) was sharply emaciated and in the region of the anterior mediastinum a solid tumour measuring 6×5×3 cm was found, protuberant and in cross section of fleshy consistency (Fig. 9).

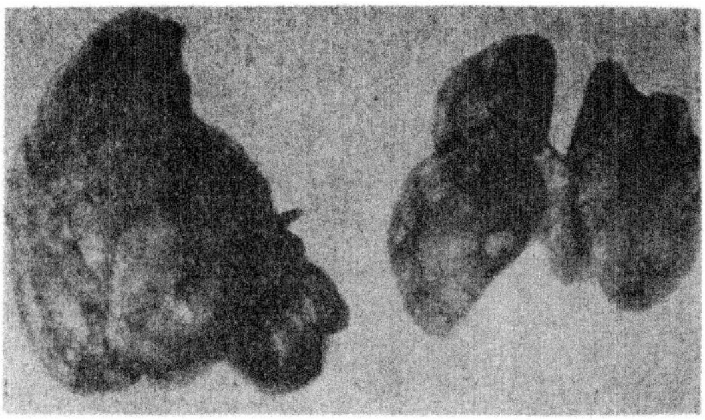

FIG. 9. Tumour in region of anterior mediastinum (rat No. 82)

Microscopic inspection revealed in the lungs of all the animals of this group moderate diffuse sclerosis and focal emphysema. Around the bronchi and in the alveolar septa accumulations of thorium were seen in the form of large chestnut-brown clumps among which there were fine layers of connective tissue, histiocytes and macrophage. The epithelium of the bronchi was succulent and peribronchially there were extensive lymphoid infiltrates. In some regional lymph nodes thorium was seen in the form of coarse dark brown clumps (not giving a reaction for iron). In the spleen there was hyperplasia of the reticulo-endothelial elements and foci of myeloid haemopoiesis were seen. In the parenchymatous organs moderate dystrophic changes were observed. In rat No. 89 the morphological changes in the lungs and organs were the same. The tumour found in the region of the mediastinum consisted of coarse, chaotically arranged connective tissue fibres in places forming continuous cicatricial fields. Here and there among the

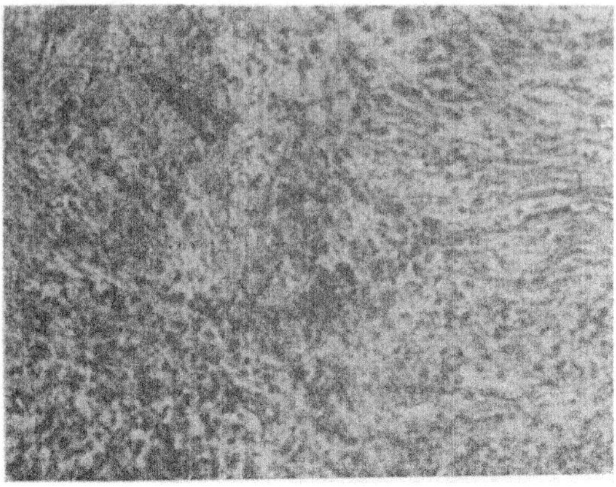

FIG. 10. Photomicrograph of tumour of right mediastinum. Bundles of chaotically arranged connective tissue fibres among which groups of atypical cells can be seen (rat No. 89). Staining with haematoxylin-eosin (×300)

fibres groups of atypical cells were encountered with misshapen nuclei and mitoses. Only in rare individual fields were remnants of lymphoid tissue seen. The tumour was of the fibrosarcoma type (Fig. 10).

After 14–15 months' exposure histological inspection of the lungs revealed moderate diffuse sclerosis, bronchiectasis with catarrhal and in places suppurative bronchitis. Around the accumulations of thorium, proliferation of connective tissue fibres could be seen with histiocytes and neutrophils among them. The epithelium of the adjacent bronchi was succulent and proliferated. In places there were the first signs of atypical development and adenomatosis. In rat No. 91, against the background of these changes, fields of necrosis and squamous cell cancer were seen with a slight tendency towards keratinization (Fig. 11).

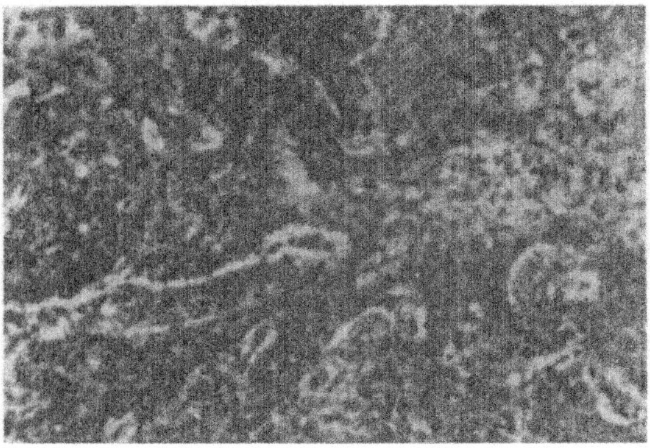

FIG. 11. Photomicrograph of lung. Islets of multi-layered squamous epithelium with onset of keratinization (rat No. 91). Staining with haematoxylin-eosin (×300)

The remaining three rats of this group died after 18–19 months' exposure. Autopsy revealed multiple abscesses of the lungs, bronchiectasis with peribronchial foci of purulent necrotic pneumonia evidently the cause of their death.

Histological inspection of the lungs showed that the further development of the pathological process proceeded by way of spread and accentuation of the chronic purulent changes with formation of multiple bronchiectasis and peribronchial inflammation of the surrounding pulmonary tissue leading in places to carnification. Nearly everywhere there was proliferation and atypical transformation of the bronchial epithelium. Two animals (Nos. 82 and 84) displayed multiple foci of bronchogenic squamous-cell keratinizing cancer of the lungs with tumour invasion into the surrounding tissues and formation of typical "pearls" with extensive areas of necrosis (Fig. 12 and 13).

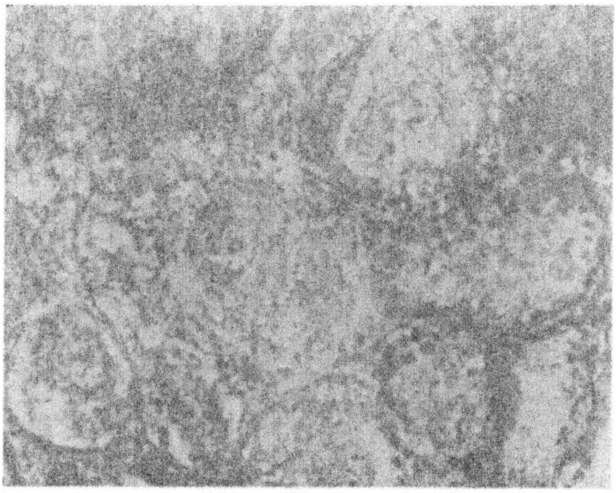

FIG. 12. Photomicrograph of lung. Honeycombs of multi-layered squamous epithelium in places with incipient keratinization (rat No. 84). Staining with haematoxylin-eosin (×300)

In the regional lymph nodes in rat No. 82 metastases of the tumour (Fig. 14) were seen and also a considerable amount of thorium. In the spleens of all the animals at this stage it was possible to observe plethora, oedema, desquamative catarrh of the sinuses and a considerable number of histiocytes, plasma cells and foci of myeloid haemopoiesis. In the liver, granular and fine droplet fatty dystrophy was observed with small focal necroses and swelling of the Kupffer cells. In the kidneys, granular dystrophy of the epithelium of the convoluted tubules was found and also focal sclerosis. In the other organs no appreciable pathological lesions were seen.

In the animals of the control group which had received a single intratracheal dose of physiological saline 6, 13, 18 and 21 months after treat-

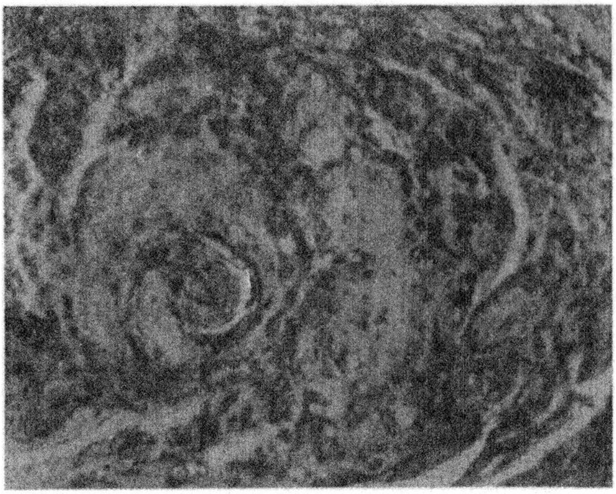

FIG. 13. Photomicrograph of lung—node of squamous cell keratinizing cancer (rat No. 82). Staining with haematoxylin-eosin (×300)

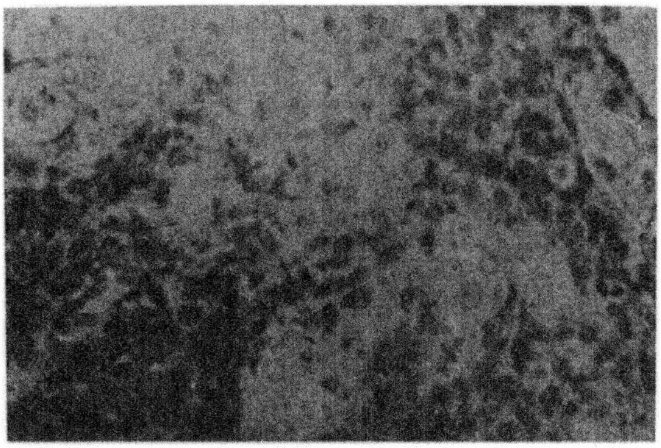

FIG. 14. Photomicrograph of bifurcation lymph node. Metastasis of squamous cell cancer (rat No. 82). Staining with haematoxylin-eosin (×300)

ment some sclerotic lesions of the pulmonary tissue related to age were identified. In some animals suppurative inflammatory phenomena were found in the lungs, and in two cases signs were found of hyperplasia of the epithelium of the bronchi and adenomatosis. No atypical cancer proliferations of the bronchial epithelium or tumours of any other localization were seen in any animal.

Thus, at various times after intratracheal administration of thorium dioxide in the test animals of all groups definite pathological lesions were demonstrated. On intratracheal administration the character of the histological pulmonary lesions was the same in all groups but their intensity varied considerably with the amount of substance administered and the time after administration.

In the animals receiving 2 mg/kg in the first 10–12 months no special morphological lesions were detected in the lungs and parenchymatous organs. With increase in the amount the thorium was distributed in the peribronchial tissue and alveolar septa. It is interesting to note that at the points of accumulation of the dust particles the cellular reaction was very slight and it was possible to see only gradually progressing sclerotic changes. In the lungs of the great majority of animals starting 13 and 21 months after treatment chronic suppurative inflammatory processes were discovered in the bronchi leading to the development of bronchiectasis and abscesses, perifocal pneumonia, adenomatosis and marked sclerotic changes of the peribronchial tissue. In addition, after 13, and particularly after 18–21 months the test animals developed tumours the number of which increased with increase in dose and times after treatment (see Table 1). The substance administered remained almost completely in the lungs and only a small fraction of it was expelled via the respiratory tract in the sputum and via the lymphatics into the regional lymph nodes where it could be detected 12–13 months after administration. In the parenchymatous organs, dystro-

TABLE 1. *Distribution of Tumours by Groups and Times of Detection*

Dose of substance administered in mg/kg	Number of animals in group	Number of animals with tumours	Times of development of tumours in months	Brief description of tumours
2	20	2	19	Cavernous angioma of the femoral region
			19	Microcellular cancer with extensive metastases
20	20	2	18	Spindle cell sarcoma of the femoral region with extensive metastases
			21	Squamous cell cancer of the lungs
200	20	3	18	Squamous cell keratinizing cancer of lungs
			19	Ditto
			21	Seminoma of the testis
300	20	4	11	Fibrosarcoma in the region of the anterior mediastinum
			14	Squamous cell keratinizing cancer of the lungs
			19	Ditto
			19	Ditto
Total	80	11(13·6%)		

phic lesions were noticed and micronecroses in the liver on high doses. We did not find any marked morphological changes in the haemopoietic organs except for haemosiderosis in the spleen which may be an indirect indicator of intensified destruction of erythrocytes.

We attach great importance to our finding that tumours develop in the lungs on intratracheal administration of ThO_2—an insoluble thorium compound. It is known that the possibility of entry of radioactive aerosols into the lungs is a very real one in conditions in which radioactive ores are obtained and enriched. However, there is a difference of opinion on the radiosensitivity of pulmonary tissue to ionizing radiations. A number of workers (Dohnert, 1938; Lorenz, 1944; and others) consider that pulmonary tissue is relatively radioresistant. Our findings, however, indicate the serious danger on entry into the lungs of an insoluble radioactive substance, which fully accords with the findings obtained previously in our laboratory by Burykina (1957), Kochetkova and Avrunina (1960) and Sagaidak (1960) in whose experiments on intratracheal administration to rats of the dioxide of radioactive ruthenium, radioactive chromium phosphate, colloidal gold and the iron-59 oxide led to the development in the animals of squamous cell keratinizing carcinoma.

Summary

1. Single intratracheal administration of thorium dioxide produces definite histological changes in the lungs and parenchymatous organs; the intensity of these changes is directly related to the dose of substance administered and the time of its action.

2. The changes in the lungs are of a uniform character and are expressed in the development of chronic suppurative lesions of the bronchi with sclerotic changes of peribronchial tissue, formation of bronchiectases, perifocal pneumonia, abscesses and adenomatous proliferations.

3. At late stages (after 13, and chiefly after 18–21 months) the test rats developed tumours (13·6 per cent)—sarcomas and squamous-cell carcinoma of the lungs. The incidence of tumours increased with increase in the dose of thorium oxide and exposure time. The minimum carcinogenic dose for the lungs on intratracheal administration was 2 mg/kg ($19{\cdot}2 \times 10^{-5}$ μCi per kg weight).

4. In the liver, changes of the protein dystrophy type were observed and in a number of cases focal micronecroses; in the kidneys, protein dystrophy of the epithelium of the convoluted tubules and in individual cases a large number of hyalin cylinders in the lumen of the tubules.

5. Distinct morphological changes and especially development of malignant tumours on admitting a single low dose of thorium oxide to the lungs

via the trachea may serve as the biological basis for stricter standardization of the maximum permissible levels of insoluble thorium compounds in the atmosphere.

References

AMORY H. I. and BUNCH R. F., Perivascular Injection of Thorotrast and its Sequelae. *Radiology*, **51**, 831–839 (1948).

BATZENSCHLAGER A., Cancer Primitif de la Travée Hépatique sur Cirrhose Thorotrastique, *Ann. Anat. Paris*, **2**, 39 (1950).

BOGLIOLO L., Spora i Blastomi Sperimentali du Ossido di Torio. *Pathologica*, **30**, 422–430 (1938).

BRODY N. and CULLEN M., Carcinoma of the Breast Seventeen Years after Mammography with Thorotrast. *Surgery*, **42**, 600–606 (1957).

BRUNNER N. E., Thorotrast Injuries. *Dtsch. med. Wschr.* **85**, 307–314 (1960).

BRUNNER N. E. and RUFTNER Y. R., Tissue Reaction of Thorium Dioxide by Peritoneal Injection. *Arch. Gewerbepath. u. Gewerbehyg.* **15**, 236–240 (1957).

BURYKINA L. N., Effect of Radioactive Ruthenium Dioxide on the Organism of White Rats Following its Intratracheal Administration. In: *The Toxicology of Radioactive Substances*, Vol. 1, pp. 139–144. Pergamon Press, Oxford (1962).

DOHNERT H. R., Experimentelle Untersuchungen zur Frage des Schneeberger Lungenkrebses. *Z. Krebsforsch.*, **47**, 209–239 (1938).

FONIO A., Über Schädigungen des Thorotrastes als Kontrastmittel. *Acta chir.* **14**, 2–29 (1947).

FOULDS L., The Production of Transplantable Carcinoma and Sarcoma in Guinea Pigs by Injections of Thorotrast. *Amer. J. Cancer*, **35**, 363–373 (1939).

GROSSIARD A., ROUCAYROL J. C., DUPERRAT B., CECCALDI P. F. and MEEUSBITH L., Adénocancer du Foie avec Cirrhose 21 Ans après une Artériographie au Thorotrast. *Bull. et mem. Soc. méd. hôp., Paris*, **72**, 49–58 (1956).

GUIMARES J. P., LAMERTON L. F. and CHRISTENSEN W. R., Late Effect of Thorotrast Administration: Review and Experimental Study. *Brit. J. Cancer*, **9**, 253 (1955).

GUSEV N. G., *Spravochnik po radioaktivnym izlucheniyam i zashchite (Reference Book on Radioactive Emanations and Protection)*. Medgiz (1956).

JOHNSEN C., Disseminated, Transmissible, Reticulo-endothelial Sarcoma in Rabbits Provoked by Intravenously Deposited Thorium. *Acta path. microbiol. Scand.*, suppl. 105, 92 (1954).

KOCHETKOVA T. A. and AVRUNINA G. A., The Long-Term Effects of Intratracheal Injection of Soluble and Insoluble Compounds of Certain Radioisotopes. In: *Toxicology of Radioactive Substances*, Vol. 2, pp. 174–185. Pergamon Press, Oxford (1963).

LORENZ E., Radioactivity and Lung Cancer: a Critical Review of Lung Cancer in the Miners of Schneeberg and Joachimsthal. *J. Nat. Cancer Inst.*, **5**, 1–45 (1944).

MCMAHON H. E. *et al.*, Endothelial-cell Sarcoma of Liver Following Thorotrast Injection. *Amer J. Path.* **23**, 585–611 (1947).

MIYAMOTO SIDEVUKI, Experimentelle Sarkomerzeugung durch Thorotrast. *Strahlentherapie*, **64**, 683–690 (1939).

MOESCHLIN S. *et al.*, Fatal Panmyelopathy due to Thorotrast. *Schweiz. med. Wschr.* **83**, 1061–1064 (1953).

MORA Y. M., Granulomatous Tumour Following Intramammary Injection of Colloidal Thorium dioxide. *J. Amer. Med. Ass.* **115**, 363–364 (1940).

NETOUŠEK M., Chronic Myelosis Following the Use of Thorotrast. *Blood*, **12**, 391 (1957).

PRUSSIA G., Contributo allo Studio dei Tumori Sperimentali di Thorotrast. *Sperimentale*, **90**, 522–539 (1936).

ROUSSY G., Action Cancerigène du Dioxyde de Thorium chez le Rat Blanc. *Bull. Acad. Med.* **112**, 809–816 (1934).

RUDOLPHI H., Spätentwicklung eines Uterinkarzinoms nach Thoriumoxydinjektion. *Beitr. path. Anat.* **111,** 158–164 (1950).

SAGAIDAK D. D., Materialy k toksikologii radioaktivnogo zheleza (The Toxicology of Radioactive Iron). Dissertation, Moscow (1960).

SELBIE, F. G. Experimental Production of Sarcoma with Thorotrast. *Lancet,* **231,** 847–848 (1936).

TARASENKO N. YU., K voprosu o toksichnosti toriya (The Toxicity of Thorium). *Gig. trud. i profzabolevanii,* **6,** 21–27 (1960).

VOGTLIN J. and MINDER W., Über Thorotrastschaden nach Bronchographie retrograder Pyelographie, Salpingographie und Arteriographie. *Radiol. Clin.* **21,** 97 (1952).

WASCHULEWSKI H., Thorotrastspeicherung und Schaden in gewerben Organen. *Dtsch. Gesundh.-Wes.* **11,** 1241 (1956).

PHOTOMETRIC DETERMINATION OF LOW AMOUNTS OF THORIUM IN BIOLOGICAL MATERIALS

N. A. PAVLOVSKAYA and T. N. CHERKASHINA

THE problem of the distribution, accumulation and elimination of thorium in biological media can be solved given sufficiently accurate, sensitive and specific methods for its determination. The methods of determining low amounts of thorium recommended in the literature do not always meet the requirements for sensitivity and specificity. Spectrometric and spectroscopic methods of determining thorium are not sensitive enough. Additional purification before spectroscopic determination complicates the method and makes its use undesirable (Hursh *et al.*, 1957; Tilton, Aldrich and Inghram, 1954; Perkins and Kalkwarf, 1956). With the emanation method proposed by Tokmakova and Turkin (1958) only radiothorium and thorium X can be determined with sufficient accuracy. The method based on extraction of thorium with mesityl oxide from liquid obtained on mineralization of the biosubstrate with subsequent turbidimetry (Belousov and Potapova, 1959) is not specific enough because titanium and zirconium interfere. Determination of thorium in the urine by means of thoron (Jeanmaire and Jammet, 1962) lacks sensitivity. A further point worth noting is that most of the methods recommended for determining thorium are intended only for analysis of urine and the use of these methods for studying organs, tissues and faeces requires additional checks.

In the search for a method for determining low amounts of thorium in biological materials we used the reagent arsenazo III proposed by Kuznetsov and Savvin (1961) for determining thorium in ores and zircons. The interaction of thorium and arsenazo III is marked by high sensitivity and selectivity. It forms with thorium a very firm emerald-green complex; with excess reagent a mixed violet colour of various hues forms.

In the view of Kuznetsov and Savvin, the reason for the formation of the unusually strong complex of thorium with arsenazo III is the non-coplanarity of the molecule and the enveloping, in space, of the ion of the element by the bent residue of the molecule.

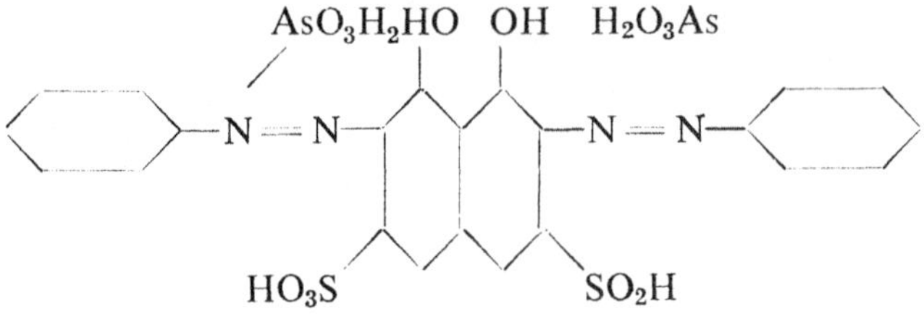

The determination of thorium with arsenazo III is impeded by Zr, Li, H, Ce and fluorides. However, the effect of most of these elements can be eliminated by adding $KMnO_4$ and ascorbic acid which results in oxidation of uranium and reduction of iron and the manganese introduced into the solution. PO_4^{3-}—in a ratio to Th of 1500 : 1—does not interfere with the determination.

To avoid the influence of zirconium 1–2 drops of 0·1 N oxalic acid are added. Fluorides greatly mask thorium but during treatment of the biological material and the liquid obtained after mineralization the fluoride is removed from solution. The sensitivity of the reaction is 0·01 γ/ml. Determination of thorium with arsenazo III is made as follows:

The biological material (muscles, internal organs, urine, faeces, blood up to 100 g) is mineralized with a mixture of sulphuric, nitric and perchloric acids, which has a number of advantages over the previously employed method of destruction by means of nitric and sulphuric acids. The time of mineralization of 100 g of the specimen is shortened from 6–8 to 1–2 hr, with a considerable reduction in the quantity of reagents used (Yablochkin). The liquid obtained after mineralization is transferred to a conical flask, diluted twice with distilled water and neutralized with 25 per cent ammonium hydroxide to pH 3 (methyl violet as indicator). The residue is filtered off, washed with 20–30 ml distilled water and dissolved in 10–20 ml 6 N HCl. Thorium is determined in the liquid obtained colorimetrically or photocolorimetrically in presence of arsenazo III.

For colorimetric determination a standard scale is prepared: into the colorimetric tubes are introduced 0·05, 0·1, 0·2, 0·4, 0·5, 0·6, 0·7, 0·8, 0·9 and 1·0 ml of the standard solution containing 10 γ Th in 1 ml 6 N HCl, then 6 N HCl is added to give 4·8 ml and then 0·2 ml of 0·05 per cent solution of arsenazo III. The test solution is prepared for colorimetry likewise. To 1–2 ml of the sample is added 6 N HCl to 4·8 ml and 0·2 ml solution of arsenazo III. If the sample is coloured yellow (presence of iron) then 5–10 ml ascorbic acid is added. The colour of the test solution is compared with the standard. To eliminate the influence of zirconium and uranium crystalline $KMnO_4$ and 1–2 drops of 0·1 N oxalic acid are added.

The amount of thorium is determined using a FEK-M photoelectrocolorimeter by means of a calibration curve obtained from the use of standard solutions. The calibration curves for thorium are presented in the figure. The determination is made on 10 ml in a cuvette at a wavelength of 680 mμ (red light filter). The test solution is prepared in the same way as for colorimetric determination. The sensitivity of the photometric determination is 0·1 γ per 5 ml. The minimum amount of thorium which can be assayed in

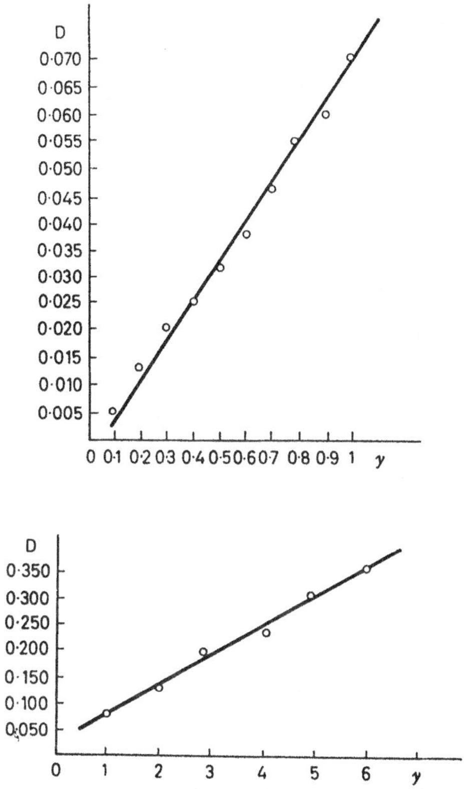

FIG. 1. Photometric determination of small amounts of thorium in biological specimens. Calibration curves for thorium: upper, 0·1–1 γ; lower, 1–6 γ

the specimen is 2 γ; the error of determination not greater than 15 per cent. The results of determination of thorium are set out in the table. A known amount of thorium in the form of $Th(NO_3)_4$ was added to the biological material and the analysis made by the method described above.

The numerals given in Table 1 are the averages for 5–8 determinations differing from the mean by not more than 5 per cent. The table indicates that determination of known amounts of thorium in such biological materials as muscle, liver, spleen and blood gives satisfactory results.

TABLE 1. *Determination of Thorium in Biological Specimens*

Ordinal number	Th γ added to biosub-strate	Thorium found in γ		
		Muscle	Liver, spleen	Blood
1	1	0·8	0·8	–
2	10	9·5	9	–
3	50	46	40	–
4	100	90	–	84
5	200	180	175	167
6	500	500	450	450
7	1000	1000	1000	920
8	Controls	0	0	0

The investigations suggest the following conclusions:

1. Thorium assay based on the reaction with arsenazo III may be used to investigate the content of small quantities of thorium in biological media.

2. The minimum determinable amount of thorium is 2γ in the sample, the error of determination is not more than 15 per cent.

3. Titanium and zirconium do not interfere with the determination. PO_4^{3-} in a ratio to Th of 1500 : 1 does not interfere with the determination.

References

BELOUSOV B. P. and POTAPOVA S. P., Determination of Low Amounts of Thorium in Biological Media (Opredeleniye malykh kolichstv toriya v biosredakh). *1958 Collection of Abstracts on Radiation Medicine*, pp. 144–145 (1959).

Determination of Thorium in the Air (Opredeleniye toriya v vozdukhe). *Collection of Radiochemical and Dosimetric Techniques (Sbornik radiokhimicheskikh i dozimetricheskikh metodik)*, pp. 139–142, Medgiz, Moscow (1959).

HURSH J. B., STEADMAN L. T., LOONEY W. B. and COLODZIN M., The Excretion of Thorium and Thorium Daughters after Thorotrast Administration. *Acta radiol.* **47**, 6, 481–498 (1957).

JEANMAIRE L. and JAMMET H., *Determination of Natural Thorium in Urine* (1962).

KUZNETSOV V. I. and SAVVIN S. V., Sensitive Photometric Determination of Thorium with the Reagent Arsenazo III (Chustvitel'noye fotometricheskoye opredeleniye toriya s reagentom arsenazo III). *Radiokhimiya*, **III**, 1, 79–86 (1961).

PERKINS R. W. and KALKWARF D. R., Determination of Thorium in Urine. *Analyt. Chem.* **28**, 12, 1989–1993 (1956).

SAVVIN S. B., Photometric Determination of Thorium and Uranium with the Reagent Arsenazo III (Fotometricheskoye opredeleniye toriya i urana s reagentom arsenazo III) *Dokl. Akad. Nauk SSSR*, **127**, 6, 1231–1234 (1959).

TILTON G. R., ALDRICH L. T. and INGHRAM M. G., Mass Spectrometric Determination of Thorium. *Analyt. Chem.* **26**, 894–898 (1954).

TOKMAKOVA YE. V. and TURKIN A. D., Determination through Thoron of Thorium X and Radiothorium in Biological Media (Opredeleniye toriya X i radiotoriya v biologicheskikh sredakh po toronu). *Meditsinskaya radiologiya*, **III**, 3, 61 (1958).

THE EFFECT OF URANOUS-URANIC OXIDE (U_3O_8) IN EXPERIMENTAL WORK

A. A. RUBANOVSKAYA

THE published findings on the toxicity of U_3O_8 are scanty and have chiefly been obtained in experiments of short duration.

Maynard and Hodge (1949) on the basis of experiments in which rats and dogs were fed for a number of months on various uranium compounds concluded that U_3O_8 is one of the weakly toxic compounds. These authors found that addition to the diet of rats of 20 per cent of uranium dioxide and uranous-uranic oxide did not retard the growth of the animals nor kill them. In the dogs only the feeding of large amounts of U_3O_8 (20 g/kg) produced minor histological changes in the liver and intestines. However, according to these workers, one dog died 17 days after oral administration of 20 g/kg U_3O_8.

Pozzani (1949) studied the toxic effect of high grade ore containing 65·8 per cent UO_2 and U_3O_8. Following inspiration of the ore dust for one month and for 4·4 hr daily at a concentration from 4·8 to 36 mg/m^3 Pozzani found that all the animal species had kidney damage varying in severity.

Wilson *et al.* (1955) allowed rabbits and rats to inhale U_3O_8 with particles of diameter of 0·5 and 2·5 μ in a dose of 80 mg/m^3 and found that the greater toxicity was shown by the particles with a diameter of 0·5 μ.

Fish (1961) reported on prolonged observation (up to 1·5 years) in persons who had accidentally inhaled U_3O_8 and also in experimental animals exposed to inhalation of this uranium compound.

We were interested in the influence on the body of prolonged administration of U_3O_8 and prolonged stay in the body of this compound. The purpose of the present investigation was to study: (1) the clinical picture of chronic poisoning with small amounts of U_3O_8 and after prolonged administration; (2) excretion of uranium in the urine and faeces and its deposition and distribution in the animal body; and (3) the pathomorphological changes in the organs of such animals.

We carried out three sets of chronic experiments in which U_3O_8 was given to the animals through the alimentary tract, the respiratory tract and under the skin. Subcutaneous administration was of interest since this enabled us to produce in the body prolonged circulation of small amounts of uranium without a local effect on pulmonary tissue and the gastro-intestinal mucosa. The substance was administered once or repeatedly during the experimental period.

Prolonged Introduction via the Gastro-intestinal Tract

The experiments were carried out on six dogs. The animals received U_3O_8 in a piece of meat 5–6 times weekly at the rate of 100 mg/kg body weight. The amount of U_3O_8 consumed by each animal in the test period was 16, 17, 22, 33 and in one case 100 g. The duration of the experiments was from one month to 50 days. During this period the dogs appeared outwardly normal, possessed a good appetite, with no change in weight in some and a slight increase in others. Urine analyses did not indicate any gross pa thology of the kidneys. In the urine we found neither albumin nor cylinders nor cellular elements.

Seven days after consumption of the last meal containing U_3O_8, the dogs were killed and a pathomorphological investigation was made. A determination was made of the uranium content of the organs and tissues. Before sacrifice (four and six days after the last administration of U_3O_8) of some dogs the uranium excreted in urine and faeces during 24 hr was measured. Determination of the content of uranium in biological media was made by the luminescent method based on fusion of uranium with sodium fluoride pearls with subsequent comparison in ultra-violet light with a standard pearl scale.

TABLE 1. *Content of Uranium in Excreta of Dogs (in mg %)*

Dog No.	4 days after last administration	6 days after last administration	
	In urine	In urine	In faeces
4	0·0024	0·002	0·7
5	0·01	0·002	0·075
6	0·0024	0·002	0·2

As Table 1 shows, excretion of uranium in the urine and faeces of the dogs occurred in very small amounts after stopping administration.

Determination of the content of uranium in the organs failed to reveal in any of the animals heavy accumulation of the metal. All the organs, apart from the kidneys and thyroid gland, contained insignificant amounts of uranium, often only traces, and in some cases it was not possible to detect even traces. In the kidneys and thyroid the amounts of uranium found exceeded its normal content in these organs. Thus, in the kidneys from 0·017 to 0·075 mg per cent was found and in the thyroid glands from 0·01 to 0·06 mg per cent.

Thus, little U_3O_8 is dissolved and absorbed in the gastro-intestinal tract. The material is almost completely removed from the gut in the first days after administration and already six days after the last administration the faeces contained only an insignificant amount of uranium.

Pathomorphological examination of the dogs revealed minor lesions in the kidneys, liver and intestines. In the kidneys here and there we noticed swelling and fatty degeneration of the tubular epithelium and in the intestinės mostly local circulatory disturbances. But all these changes had no effect on the general condition of the animals throughout the observation period.

Introduction of U_3O_8 into the Trachea

Experiments on rabbits. In all, 32 rabbits were used (28 test animals and 4 controls). A single dose of U_3O_8 in the form of a suspension in saline was injected by puncture of the inferior trachea. The control rabbits received saline by the same route. The amount of fluid introduced was 1·5–2 ml and the amount of U_3O_8 was 100–300 mg (30–120 mg/kg).

Seventeen animals (13 test, 4 controls) were under observation from 3 to 10·5 months, six rabbits were killed 4–9 days and nine rabbits 2·5 months after administration.

With the route of administration employed by us it would appear that not all the substance introduced reached the pulmonary tissue and was consequently not retained in the lungs. It may be assumed that some of it settled on the mucosa of the trachea and in the lumen of the bronchi from where it was rapidly removed. To clear up this problem six rabbits were killed in the days following administration of U_3O_8 and its content in the lungs determined.

The determinations showed that 4–9 days after intratracheal administration of U_3O_8 the lungs contained 53–79 per cent of the amount administered. It was of interest to clarify the subsequent fate of this material retained in the lung. For this purpose nine rabbits were killed 2·5 months after poisoning and the lung content of U_3O_8 determined (Table 3).

Table 3 shows that 2·5 months after administration of 200–220 mg/kg U_3O_8, 53 per cent of the dose given remained in the lungs in only one case. In the lungs of the other rabbits the amount found was considerably less than in the first few days after administration. Thus, the amount of U_3O_8 in the lungs falls with time.

TABLE 2. *Content of* U_3O_8 *in Lungs of Rabbits 4–9 Days after Intratracheal Administration*

Rabbit No.	Injected in mg	Time after injection in days	Found	
			In mg	% of amount given
1	100	4	54·35	54·35
2	200	4	106	63
3	200	4	117·6	58·7
4	200	4	118	58·8
5	300	9	189·3	63·1
6	300	9	234	79

TABLE 3. *Content of* U_3O_8 *in Lungs of Rabbits 2·5 Months after Intratracheal Administration*

Rabbit No.	U_3O_8 injected in mg	U_3O_8 found	
		In mg	% of amount given
7	220	88·75	40·34
8	220	88·75	40·34
9	220	117·16	53·45
10	200	59·17	29·59
11	200	71·00	35·5
12	200	29·58	14·79
13	200	59·17	29·59
14	200	88·75	41·38
15	200	88·75	44·38

Of the 15 test rabbits kept under prolonged observation two died 100 days after administration of U_3O_8. Autopsy in one case revealed unresolved pregnancy and, in another, pneumonia. The other rabbits were killed after 5·5 to 10·5 months. During the test period an observation was kept on the general state of the animals and their weight. The excretion of uranium in the urine and faeces was periodically checked. The organs of the killed animals were analysed for content of uranium and inspected histologically. Outwardly, the test rabbits did not differ from normal controls. During the first 10 days after administration of the material the rabbits lost weight, then the weight was rapidly restored and subsequently increased (116–132 per cent of the original).

For many months after administration of U_3O_8 small amounts of uranium were found in the urine and faeces of the rabbits. Starting from the second month after administration of 100–120 mg of uranium per kg of body weight the amount in a 24-hr sample of urine and faeces varied in the different periods of observation from traces to 0·13 mg per cent. After administration of 30–50 mg/kg the corresponding amounts were from 0 to 0·25 mg per cent. Excretion of uranium was not uniform and in most of the rabbits a fall became obvious with time. This was related to a reduction in the amount of U_3O_8 in the lungs and to a change in the distribution of the particles.

Together with removal of particles of the material from the lungs there was also another process which tended to retain particles. Morphological examination of the lungs showed that the particles of U_3O_8 which were initially distributed diffusely tended to form with time large compact round conglomerations in the lymphoid tissue. These were sometimes encircled by thin bands of connective tissue. On formation of these nodes the particles were fixed and retained in the lungs. With the formation of such solid conglomerations the surface of contact between particles and tissue fluid became smaller. This apparently changed the conditions of transfer of the particles of uranous-uranic oxide from the lungs and was one of the causes of reduced excretion from the body.

The intensity of these two processes undoubtedly varied from animal to animal and, therefore, many months after administration of identical doses the lungs of some rabbits contained different amounts of U_3O_8.

As stated above, in the rabbits killed at late times the content of U_3O_8 was determined in the lungs and other tissues and organs. Table 4 shows that from 5·5 to 10·5 months after administration the amount of U_3O_8 remaining in the lungs of the rabbits was smaller than after 2·5 months, its amount varying within fairly narrow limits; from 5·5 to 19·3 per cent

TABLE 4. *Content of* U_3O_8 *in Lungs of Rabbits 5·5–10·5 Months after Intratracheal Administration*

Rabbit No.	U_3O_8 injected in mg	Times after injection	U_3O_8 found	
			In mg	% of amount given
16	270	10 months 22 days	15	5.55
17	110	10 months 15 days	20	18·2
18	110	10 months 15 days	15·7	14·3
19	270	9 months 15 days	24·2	9
20	140	8 months 10 days	27	19·3
21	100	8 months 10 days	19	19
22	110	8 months 10 days	16	14·5
23	100	8 months 10 days	7·2	6
24	300	5 months 15 days	76·9	25·6
25	300	5 months 15 days	41·4	13·8

of that administered. After 5·5 months the lungs of only one rabbit contained 25·6 per cent of the amount of U_3O_8 administered. Evidently, at the end of a certain period, the process of removal of particles of the compound from the lungs of the rabbit practically ceased.

Determination of the content of uranium in the organs of the rabbits at the end of the experiment (after 8·5–10·5 months) showed that all the organs contained insignificant amounts of uranium, often only traces. Sometimes it was not possible to find uranium in certain organs. The content was highest in the kidneys where we found from 0·023 to 0·12 mg per cent uranium (Table 5).

TABLE 5. *Content of Uranium (in mg %) in Rabbit Organs 8·5–10·5 Months after Intratracheal Administration*

Rabbit No.	21	20	18	17	19	16
U_3O_8 introduced in mg	100	140	110	110	270	270
Observation period, months	$8^1/_2$	$8^1/_2$	$10^1/_2$	$10^1/_2$	$9^1/_2$	$10^1/_2$
Test organs:						
Suprarenals	0·055	0·08	0·01	—	—	0
Lymph nodes (mesenterial)	0·0083	0·005	0·028	—	0·05	0·0055
Bone marrow	0·02	0·004	—	—	0·06	0·066
Spleen	0·0081	0·14	0·009	—	0·061	0·028
Heart	0·007	0·0035	0·002	—	0	0·0025
Brain	0	0·0022	0·001	0·003	0·002	0·005
Liver	0·003	0·06	0·01	0·017	0·033	0·00
Large intestine	0·0023	0·0017	0·0085	0·005	0·033	0·00
Small intestines	0·0071	0·002	0·0005	0·0027	0·033	0·00
Kidneys	0·066	0·036	0·023	0·081	0·12	0·07
Sex glands	0·021	—	0·011	—	0·013	0·00
Blood	0	0	0	0	0	0
Urine	0·0042	0·003	0	0·023	0·01	0·004
Lungs	—	225	178	—	224	150

Comparison of the findings for the rabbits killed at 10·5 months and at shorter intervals shows that the content of uranium in the organs did not increase with lengthening of the period of sojourn. For prolonged stay of U_3O_8 in the lungs, the accumulation of uranium in other organs apart from kidney was not heavy.

Thus, the experiments showed that U_3O_8 in the lungs for 10·5 months had no effect on the general condition of the rabbits, which remained outwardly normal and put on weight, but somewhat less than in the normal controls.

However, morphological investigations revealed a number of lesions in the organs of these rabbits. They are described in the work of Tolgskaya (this volume, pp. 120–135).

Experiments on dogs. The suspension of U_3O_8 was introduced into the trachea of dogs in a single dose by means of a throat syringe. The technique of administration was as follows. The dogs were lightly anaesthetized (intravenous injection of a minimum anaesthetic dose of hexenal with anaesthesia of the mucosa of the larynx and the trachea with cocaine). The animals did not cough for some time and therefore, much of the compound had time to settle in the lung tissue.

In three dogs killed four days after intratracheal administration by this method we found in the lungs of dog No. 1 given 1 g of U_3O_8 0·35 g (35 per cent), in dog No. 2 (given 0·6 g) 0·186 g (31 per cent) and in dog No. 3 (given 0·6 g) 0·228 g (38 per cent). Thus, we may tentatively consider that in the dogs with this route of administration from 31 to 38 per cent of the amount of U_3O_8 given is retained in the lungs.

Ten dogs were given a single dose of 0·3 to 1 g U_3O_8: six dogs 70–100 mg per kg weight and four dogs 30–50 mg/kg. Introduction into the lungs of these amounts of the compound produced acute poisoning characterized by the same signs as for soluble uranium salts. It must be stated that U_3O_8 used in this series of experiments was somewhat more finely dispersed than that in the experiments on rabbits.

During the 10–12 days after administration of the compound a picture of severe kidney damage developed. In the blood there was a sharp rise in non-protein nitrogen (up to 350 mg per cent and in one case one day before death 600 mg per cent) with appearance in the urine of albumin, hyaline cylinders and a large number of leucocytes. The dogs lost appetite and subsequently refused all food, vomited and rapidly lost weight; some died, the others gradually recovered. Of the six dogs given intratracheally from 70–100 mg/kg, two died one 10 and one 11 days after administration. Of the four dogs given 30–50 mg/kg two died, one 10 days and one 20 days after administration.

In the surviving dogs 1·5 months after administration, non-protein nitrogen in the blood and the composition of the urine approached normal and body weight was restored (Table 6). The dogs which survived acute poisoning were kept under observation for different periods. Two dogs were killed at 2 months 5 days, one at 5·5 months, one at 8 months and

TABLE 6. *Changes in Body Weight. Non-protein Nitrogen in the Blood and Composition of Urine in Dogs after Acute Poisoning with* U_3O_8

U_3O_8 introduced in mg	Dog No. 1					Dog No. 2					Dog No. 5					Dog No. 7				
	800					800					400					700				
Times after administration of U_3O_8 in days	Weight in kg	Non-protein nitrogen in mg per cent	Urine in ‰	Leucocytes in urine per field of vision	Hyaline cylinders per field of vision	Weight in kg	Non-protein nitrogen in mg per cent	Urine in ‰	Leucocytes in urine per field of vision	Hyaline cylinders per field of vision	Weight in kg	Non-protein nitrogen in mg per cent	Urine in ‰	Leucocytes in urine per field of vision	Hyaline cylinders per field of vision	Weight in kg	Non-protein nitrogen in mg per cent	Urine in ‰	Leucocytes in urine per field of vision	Hyaline cylinders per field of vision
0 (before poisoning)	12	38				10	31·5				13	25				9·5	40			
2												60	0·33	50	0–1					0–1
7												110	0·66	40–60	0–1		210	0·3	20–40	
9–10	10·1	300				7·7	600				11·5	80				7·6	350			
20						Died after 10 days						40				Died after 11 days				
32	9·8	80	0·16	15–20	0–1															
41–47	10·4	40	Traces	3–5	None						13		Traces	20–30	0–1					
150	12·6																			

TABLE 7. *Content of Uranium in Urine and Faeces of Dogs at Various Times after Acute Poisoning with* U_3O_8 *(in mg %)*

Dog No.	1		3		4		5		9		10	
Introduced in mg	800		800		600		400		800		1000	
Times after poisoning in days	Urine	Faeces	Urine	Faeces	Urine	Faeces	Urine	Faeces	Urine	Faeces	Urine	Faeces
2	0·035	60·0	0·05	—	0·065	—	0·085	—	—	—	—	—
4–5	0·07	—	0·03	—	0·015	0·70	0·025	—	—	—	0·0045	—
7–10	0·015	—	0·05	—	0·017	—	0·015	0·04	0·006	—	—	—
16–21	0·015	—	0·0045	—	0·007	—	0·017	0	—	—	—	—
30	0·04	0·06	0·0012	0·02	—	—	—	—	—	—	0·015	—
40					0·002	0	0·007	0	0·005			
50–60	0·004	0	0·004	0·01			0·002	0				
65–70					0	0	0·002	0	0·03	0·010	0·002	0·024
90	0·002	0	0·0018	0					0·032	0·02	0·002	0
110–150	0·015	0	0	0					0·003	0		
200	0·01	0							0·007	0		
205–240	0	0							0·0005	0	0	0
285												

two at 9·5 months after poisoning. Throughout the observation period we made periodic checks on urinary uranium and its content in separate portions of faeces. The results are presented in Table 7.

As was also observed in the rabbits, uranium was excreted from the dogs in the urine and faeces. Only in the first few days after poisoning did the faeces contain a considerable amount of uranium. This was the part of the U_3O_8 transported from the lungs to the throat and eliminated from the body via the gut. Subsequently, uranium excreted in the faeces settled at a low level in the range of 0·01–0·06 mg per cent. With time the excretion of uranium in the faeces ceased.

The content of uranium in the urine in the first days after poisoning varied from 0·035 to 0·085 mg per cent and then fell to 1000ths of a mg per cent and subsequently to zero. Thus, after severe acute poisoning with U_3O_8 the excretion of uranium in the urine and faeces ceased with time. Our determinations did not give an exhaustive picture of the course of excretion of uranium in the urine and faeces since these determinations were made periodically. The results afford an idea of the pathways and duration of excretion of uranium after intratracheal administration.

Determination of the content of U_3O_8 in the lungs of dogs at the end of the experiments showed that in this organ only an insignificant part of the amount given remained (Table 8).

TABLE 8. *Content of U_3O_8 in Lungs of Dogs at Various Times after Acute Poisoning*

Dog No.	U_3O_8 introduced in mg	Times after administration in days	U_3O_8 found	
			In mg	% of amount given
4	600	65	2·96	0·49
5	400	65	10·06	2·52
3	800	165	4·14	0·52
1	800	240	10·06	1·33
9	800	285	9·47	1·19
10	1000	285	3	0·31

Table 8 shows that after 65 days the lungs contained only 0·5–2·5 per cent of the amount of U_3O_8 administered. Roughly the same amounts were found in the dogs alive 240–285 days after poisoning (0·3–1·3 per cent). Evidently, removal of the bulk of the compound from the lungs occurs in the early stages after poisoning.

From the published findings it is known that on poisoning of animals with soluble uranium compounds pneumonia is observed in a large number of cases. Evidently, the compound introduced into the lungs is swiftly removed in the catarrhal secretion of the alveoli and bronchi. In rabbits 5·5–10·5 months after administration more U_3O_8 remained in the lungs than in dogs. The greater retention of the compound in the lungs of rabbits was due to formation of compact conglomerations in the lymphoid tissue in the form of solid nodes, formations not found in the lungs of the dogs.

The above-described gradual reduction in the elimination of uranium in this group of dogs was connected with reduction in the amount of U_3O_8 in the lungs. Determination of the content of uranium in the organs of these dogs showed that most of it was contained in the kidneys and some in the liver (Table 9). Some organs contained no uranium at all in a number

TABLE 9. *Content of Uranium in Organs of Dogs at Various Times after Poisoning with* U_3O_8 (*in mg* %)

Dog No.	4	5	3	1	9	10
Times after burdening in days	65	65	165	240	285	285
Organs:						
Thyroid	0·01	0	0·022	0·009	0·017	0·011
Spleen	0·005	0·0025	0·0025	0·01	0	0·0025
Pancreas	0	0	0	0	0·002	0·005
Brain	0	0	0	0	0·0025	0·0025
Liver	0·002	0·035	0·006	0·05	0·050	0·025
Muscles	—	0	0	0	0	0
Testes	0·0032	0·0016	0·015	0	—	—
Ovaries	—	—	—	0	0	0·0091
Large intestine	0·02	—	—	0	0·002	0·035
Small intestines	0	0	0	0	0	0·01
Kidneys	0·07	0·12	0·12	0·1	0·08	0·05
Bone	0	0	—	0	0	0
Bronchial glands	22·2	14	—	—	—	—
Lungs	2·7	8·4	6·9	12	14·6	3·3

of cases. Consequently, the series of experiments carried out on dogs showed that U_3O_8 is vigorously removed from the lungs until they are almost completely cleared of the particles. In line with this with time there is reduction and then arrest of elimination of uranium.

Similar findings were obtained by Fish (1961). According to the observations of this author the lungs of a person who inhaled U_3O_8 by accident contained after 1·5 years about 3 per cent of the original amount of uranium.

In our experiments on dogs which were subjected to severe poisoning with U_3O_8, when 3–10 mg of the compound was found in the lungs 0 to 0·002 mg per cent uranium was recovered in the urine. Uranium in the organs varied from 0 to 0·12 mg per cent.

The pathomorphological investigation showed changes in the kidneys, lungs, lymph nodes and spleen of the same nature as in the rabbits given U_3O_8 intratracheally. These changes are discussed in detail in the paper by Tolgskaya (this volume, pp. 120–135).

Subcutaneous Administration of U_3O_8 in Rabbits

As stated at the beginning of this paper, by introducing under the skin a certain amount of U_3O_8 we endeavoured to bring about prolonged circulation in the body of small constant amounts of uranium. The test animals were rabbits.

The subcutaneously injected U_3O_8 lies in a compact mass under the skin and the surface of contact with the tissue fluid was thus very limited. Uranium from the injection site must dissolve and be absorbed into the body to a much lesser extent than in the lungs. Therefore, we introduced under the skin comparatively large amounts of U_3O_8 of 1–1·4 g and 0·5–0·7 g/kg body weight. Two rabbits were given much larger quantities — 3·5 and 2·5 g per animal. U_3O_8 was introduced under the skin in a small amount of saline in doses of 0·2–0·25 g. The compound was introduced 5–6 times at intervals of 10–14 days, the duration of the experiments was 7 months. The experiment was carried out on 17 rabbits, of which four died after 3–5 months from supervening infection (pneumonia, etc.). The other rabbits remained outwardly normal and put on weight. No skin lesions at the site of administration and deposition of the product were found nor were there any necroses or falling out of the hair. Increase in the weight of the animals during the observation period was as much as 45 per cent of the original. Only two rabbits given subcutaneously 2·5 and 3·5 g showed a considerable weight loss at the end of the experiment (21·8 and 41 per cent of the initial weight); both animals were in a poor state when killed.

Six weeks after the end of the subcutaneous injections of U_3O_8 several repeat determinations of the content of uranium in the urine were made in some rabbits. The determinations were made on the urine of five rabbits each receiving subcutaneously 1 g and on the urine of one rabbit given 3·5 g of the compound. The urine was investigated three times on different days at intervals of two days.

Table 10 shows that in all the rabbits examined uranium was found in the urine and with presence under the skin of 3·5 g U_3O_8 the content of uranium in the urine was greater than for a content of 1 g of the compound.

TABLE 10. *Content of Uranium in Urine of Rabbits 1·5 Months after Subcutaneous Injection of* U_3O_8

Rabbit No.	Amount injected subcutaneously in g	Found in urine at various times in mg %
1	1	0·0006
2	1	0·0004–0·0008
3	1	0·005–0·015
4	1	0·0014–0·02
5	1	0·002–0·03
6	3·5	0·08–0·1

Determination of the uranium content of the organs of rabbits of this group revealed in the main the same distribution as in the first two series of experiments. The amount of uranium in all the organs apart from the kidneys varied approximately within the same limits as in the rabbits with considerably smaller amounts of U_3O_8 in the lungs.

Our findings show that prolonged circulation of small amounts of uranium causes certain morphological changes in the internal organs of rabbits although the animals remained virtually normal during an observation period of seven months. Only in the two rabbits given 2·5 and 3·5 g did a picture of severe intoxication develop at the end of the experiment.

Summary

1. The introduction into the canine gastro-intestinal tract for 30–50 days of considerable amounts of U_3O_8 (17, 33 and 100 g) did not influence the general state of health of the animals. The compound was almost completely removed in the faeces. The substance did not dissolve in the gastro-intestinal tract and was consequently only absorbed to a very limited degree. Histological inspection of the organs indicated only a minor degenerative process in the kidneys and local disturbances in blood circulation in the intestinal wall.

2. Single introduction into the lungs of considerable amounts of U_3O_8 (up to 1 g) produced severe intoxication in dogs.

3. The particles of U_3O_8 were vigorously removed from the lungs through the air passages, a considerable proportion of them entering the regional lymph nodes. The bulk of the product was removed from the lungs in the early stages after poisoning. Some particles removed from the lungs were swallowed and excreted in the faeces. Formation in the lymphoid tissue of compact conglomerations of U_3O_8 resulted in less vigorous removal in the rabbit than in the dogs.

4. Rabbits in which 7·2 to 76·9 mg of U_3O_8 was found at death had remained virtually normal for 5·5–10·5 months. However, morphological examination showed a minor degenerative process in the kidney and a chronic interstitial process in the lungs with accumulation of the product in the form of compact demarcated nodes.

5. The dogs which survived severe intoxication with U_3O_8 subsequently remained outwardly normal and put on weight. The morphological changes in the kidneys and lungs were of the same nature as in the rabbits.

6. A depot under the skin of considerable amounts of U_3O_8 (1 and 1·4 g per rabbit) for seven months had no toxic effect and except for the kidneys did not lead to accumulation of uranium in the organs. Pathological lesions in the organs were weakly marked. On subcutaneous administration of 2·5–3·5 g U_3O_8 severe intoxication developed.

References

Fish B. R., Inhalation of Uranium Aerosols by Mouse, Rat, Dog and Man. In: *Inhaled Particles and Vapours.* Proceedings of an International Symposium (Editor Davies, C. N.), Pergamon Press (1961).

Haven F. L., Tolerance to Uranium Compounds. In: *Pharmacology and Toxicology of Uranium Compounds,* Vol. 1, pp. 729–758 (Editors Voegtlin C. and Hodge H. C.). McGraw-Hill, New York (1949).

Maynard E. A. and Hodge H. C., Studies of Toxicity of Various Uranium Compounds when Fed to Experimental Animals. In: *Pharmacology and Toxicology of Uranium Compounds,* Vol. I, pp. 309–376 (Editors Voegtlin C. and Hodge H. C.). McGraw-Hill, New York (1949).

McNider W., Functional and Pathological Response of Kidney in Dogs Subjected to Second Subcutaneous Injection of Uranium Nitrate. *J. Exp. Med.* **49,** 411–433 (1929).

McNider W., Acquired Resistance of Fixed Tissue Cells to Chemical Injury. *South Med. J.* **29,** 1189–1194 (1936).

Pozzani U. C., High-grade Ores. In: *Pharmacology and Toxicology of Uranium Compounds,* Vol. I, pp. 622–635 (Editors Voegtlin C. and Hodge H. C.). McGraw-Hill New York (1949).

Stokinger H. E., Rothenstein A., Roberts E., Spiegl C. J., Dygert H. P., La Belle C. W. and Sprague G. F., Toxicity following Inhalation. In: *Pharmacology and Toxicology of Uranium Compounds,* Vol. I, pp. 423–524 (Editors Voegtlin C. and Hodge H. C.). McGraw-Hill, New York (1949).

Wilson H. B., Sylvester G. E., Laskin S., La Belle C. W., Scott J. K. and Stokinger H. E., Relation of Particle Size of U_3O_8 Dust to Toxicity Following Inhalation by Animals. *Arch. Indust. & Hlth.* **11,** 11 (1955).

Woroshilsky Y., Wirkung des Urans. Thesis, Dorpat (1889).

CHANGES IN THE PERIPHERAL BLOOD FOLLOWING CHRONIC AND ACUTE POISONING WITH U_3O_8

N. L. BELOBORODOVA

THE majority of investigations concerned with the toxicology of uranium have concentrated on the effect on the body of the readily soluble nitrate, while the insoluble or poorly soluble compounds including uranous-uranic oxide (U_3O_8) have received little attention. The toxicity of U_3O_8 was studied in greater detail by the staff of the pharmacological department of the Manhattan project, U.S.A., whose results were published in the collection *Pharmacology and Toxicology of Uranium Compounds* (1949).

Investigation of the effect of U_3O_8 for different routes of administration showed that its application to the skin in the form of 65 per cent suspension does not produce in animals any signs of intoxication whereas application of soluble salts may result in death (Orcutt, 1949).

As noted by Maynard and Hodge (1949), symptoms of poisoning are absent after administration to rats of 20 per cent U_3O_8 in the food. These workers showed in other experiments that a dog given U_3O_8 by mouth in an amount of 20 g/kg daily died on the 17th day with signs of damage to the kidneys, liver and gastro-intestinal tract typical of uranium. The maximum tolerated dose of U_3O_8 is put by these workers at 10 g/kg animal weight. Here, the dog did not die for a month but the authors indicate that this dose undoubtedly is too high in view of the high sensitivity of dogs to uranium. Investigation of the toxicity of U_3O_8 by inhalation showed that this compound gives a characteristic picture of intoxication in various animal species for an air content of 17–20 mg/m^3 (Stokinger *et al.*, 1949).

The published findings mentioned indicate that the toxicity of U_3O_8 as compared with soluble uranium compounds is relatively low.

Change in the morphological composition of the blood was only found after inhalation of high doses (20 mg/m^3) uranyl nitrate. Twenty-four hours after exposure rats were found to have a reduced red cell count, haemoglobin and lymphocytes. In rabbits, an increase in the number of thrombocytes, leucocytes and neutrophils was noted (Stokinger *et al.*, 1949).

Unfortunately, in the papers mentioned the figures obtained for the blood analyses are not indicated nor is the duration of the observations stated. There is complete absence of haematological investigations for chronic exposure. In view of this we investigated changes in the blood for different routes of administration of U_3O_8 in acute and chronic experiments on dogs given the material by mouth and via the trachea. Before the start of poisoning and also systematically during the experiment haematological investigations were carried out: overall clinical analysis of the blood, reticulocyte count and also cytology by the method of Professor A. P. Yegorov. The same investigations were carried out on control dogs.

Changes in the Peripheral Blood after Oral Administration of U_3O_8

The investigation was carried out on eight dogs given U_3O_8 in a piece of cooked meat 5–6 times weekly at the rate of 100 mg/kg. Throughout the experimental period the dogs received 16, 17, 22, 33 and 100 g.

No deviations from normal were observed in the red blood indices in the test dogs. The total number of leucocytes changed irregularly but with a tendency to increase to the upper limit of normal. In all the dogs by the 3rd–4th month of the experiment we noted a certain rise in the absolute lymphocyte count from 2500 to 4200 per mm^3 and for monocytes from 300 to 860 per mm^3 (Tables 1 and 2). All the animals were in good shape.

Three dogs were killed for histological inspection and determination of the uranium content of the organs. Three more of the dogs were given U_3O_8 intratracheally.

The morphological investigations carried out by Tolgskaya (this volume, pp. 120–135) showed that gross organ lesions were absent in these animals. The histological changes in the liver and kidneys were slight. In the spleen and lymph nodes there was some hyperplasia of the reticulo-endothelium without reduction in lymphoid elements.

Changes in the Peripheral Blood after Intratracheal Administration of U_3O_8

The intratracheal mode of administration of U_3O_8 in dogs was employed in two sets of experiments. In the first, low doses of U_3O_8 were repeatedly administered not producing visible symptoms of intoxication and in the second, U_3O_8 was given as a single dose producing acute poisoning.

The changes in the peripheral blood after repeat intratracheal administration of U_3O_8 in low doses. Because of the similar results we put into this group seven dogs of which three (Nos. 1, 2 and 3) before intratracheal administration had received U_3O_8 in the food. No symptoms of intoxication were observed in this period. They ate well and put on weight. In respect of the peripheral blood they differed from the control dogs only in somewhat higher absolute lymphocyte and monocyte counts (Tables 1 and 2).

The other four dogs were given U_3O_8 only via the trachea. The control dogs received saline by the same route. U_3O_8 was given with a throat syringe in the form of a suspension every 15–20 days for 2 months to a total of 0·3–0·5 g of U_3O_8 per kg of animal weight. However, part of the substance was expelled to the exterior by coughing, as found by Rubanovskaya (this volume, p. 93), and 5·5–8·5 per cent of the dose given remained in the lungs, or 0·01–0·02 g/kg animal weight. As shown by urine analyses the dogs excreted thousandths of a milligram of uranium.

TABLE 1. *Absolute Numbers of Individual Types of Leucocytes per* mm^3 *following Oral and Intratracheal Administration of* U_3O_8 *in Dog No. 1*

Date	Total number of leucocytes	Neutrophils	Eosinophils	Lymphocytes	Monocytes	Notes
1st year of experiment						
February	7 700	4543	308	2541	308	Before poisoning
March	8 320	4814	415	2656	415	Poisoning by mouth
April	12,000	6480	600	3840	600	
May	12,000	6954	366	4270	611	
June	10,720	6000	360	3800	560	
July	12,150	7260	726	3630	484	Poisoning via the trachea
August	12,000	8040	180	4560	300	
September	18,000	9540	360	7200	900	
October	9 750	5626	582	3201	291	
November	9 500	6650	522	2565	142	
December	9 100	5842	591	1911	728	
2nd year of experiment						
January	7 975	6000	79	1200	632	
February	5 800	4292	232	609	377	
March	6 200	4402	372	1023	372	
April	7 075	3570	1190	1120	385	
May	7 750	4081	1771	1078	654	
June	9 500	4845	1520	2185	855	
July	9 325	5952	1209	1767	279	

TABLE 2. *Absolute Numbers of Individual Types of Leucocytes per mm³ following Oral and Intratracheal Administration of* U_3O_8 *in Dog No. 2*

Date	Total number of leucocytes	Neutrophils	Eosinophils	Lymphocytes	Monocytes	Notes
1st year of experiment						
February	10,600	7 526	424	2544	318	Before poisoning
March	8 750	4 872	318	2610	435	Poisoning by mouth
April	10,530	5 775	787	3150	778	
May	12,400	6 820	868	3968	774	
June	14,520	8 700	870	4060	870	
July	17,750	10,620	1127	5310	531	Poisoning via the trachea
August	15,380	8 415	1021	5056	918	
September	15,200	8 360	1216	4560	1064	
October	17,500	11,462	875	4725	350	
November	13,950	9 313	903	3614	139	
December .	18,100	12,966	362	3620	2172	
2nd year of experiment						
January	23,650	18,408	354	2382	2365	
February	16,400	9 676	2460	2460	1722	
March	13,200	8 580	1386	2310	927	
April	11,300	7 232	791	2260	1017	
May	13,000	9 030	585	2210	910	
June	12,750	8 980	444	2603	762	
July	13,000	7 415	1560	2600	1235	
August	15,675	11,700	152	1950	1950	

The animals of this group were under observation for 7–12 months and when killed were in a good general condition. Blood analyses were made once a month. The changes in the peripheral blood were quite similar in all seven dogs. The red blood composition showed no special changes. The count per thousand of reticulocytes was about 5–8. The leucocyte count changed in wavelike fashion and in individual periods we observed moderate neutrophilic leucocytosis.

The most characteristic feature was a fall in the absolute number of lymphocytes in all dogs with periodically monocytosis and eosinophilia.

The dogs which had received U_3O_8 by mouth had a somewhat higher initial level of absolute lymphocyte count and the reduction did not start immediately after going over to intratracheal administration (Tables 1 and 2).

The cytology of the leucocytes in this group of dogs showed considerable deviations from normal with an increase in the number of neutrophils which displayed fragmentation of the nucleus to differing degrees ranging from incipient (in the form of "thorns" and "whiskers") to complete splitting off of small pieces of the nucleus. In some cases the number of neutrophils with a fragmented nucleus reached 20 per cent and higher which, according to the findings of Professor A. P. Yegorov, indicates disturbance in the early phases of mitosis of the neutrophils in the bone marrow.

The number of disintegrating cells (cytolysis) was also somewhat raised and reached 8–10 per cent as against 2–3 per cent before the start of poisoning with U_3O_8. Changes in the nuclei of the lymphocytes and monocytes were observed in the form of vacuolization and fragmentation.

In line with the lymphopenia observed by us and the degenerative changes in the nuclei of the lymphocytes on histological inspection of the organs of the dogs of this group Tolgskaya (this volume, pp. 120–135) found depletion of lymphoid elements in the spleen, lymph nodes and pulmonary lymph follicles. Often the lymphocyte nuclei were damaged (karyorrhexis). In the dogs given repeated amounts of U_3O_8 via the trachea we observed some disturbance in neutrophil leucopoiesis and changes in lymphopoiesis. These changes were accompanied by morphological changes in the lymphoid tissue, changes not reflected in the general state of the dogs, which were in a good condition when killed.

Single acute poisoning. To study the picture of the peripheral blood in acute poisoning three dogs (Nos. 8, 9 and 10) were given U_3O_8 (80 mg/kg) via the trachea under shallow general hexenal anaesthesia with use of local anaesthesia of the mucosa of the larynx and trachea with cocaine.

The symptoms of intoxication began to appear from the 5th–6th day and reached their peak on the 9th–10th day. The dogs gradually stopped taking food, weakened and became sharply emaciated losing as much as 20 per cent of their initial weight with development of a typical picture of acute nephrosis: a large amount of albumin (up to 6·6 ‰) was found in the urine plus hyaline cylinders.

In the blood there was sharp increase in non-protein nitrogen: dog No. 8 which died on the 10th day gave a figure of 600 mg. In the two surviving dogs (Nos. 10 and 9) the symptoms of intoxication differed in intensity. Dog No. 10 was in a relatively good condition while dog No. 9 displayed very severe intoxication.

The changes in the peripheral blood in all three dogs were roughly of the same nature. On the days when the condition of the dogs was particularly severe we observed increase in the red cell count (on average by 2,000,000 per mm^3) and haemoglobin (by 15–20 per cent). It appears that this was due to blood coagulation setting in during this period, since the dogs refused food and water. In the two surviving dogs, erythrocyte counts and haemoglobin rapidly returned to normal.

With the developing picture of intoxication there was a sharp fall in polychromasia and disappearance from the blood of reticulocytes which indicates depression of erythropoiesis.

On the 9th–12th days the dogs developed neutrophilic leucocytosis reaching high values (20,000–30,000 per mm^3). In the nuclear formula of the neutrophils we at first noted a shift to the right, then in the dogs which withstood poisoning a shift to the left.

In all the dogs at this period the absolute and relative numbers of lymphocytes sharply fell to 1–2 per cent of normal (147–400 cells per mm^3 blood). Eosinophils disappeared from the blood for a certain period. At the same time, we observed absolute and relative monocytosis especially sharply marked in the presence of severe intoxication. Together with the shift to the right in the nuclear formula of the neutrophils, cytological changes appeared in the leucocytes. A large number of neutrophils showed fragmentation of the nucleus (12–25 per cent), the monocytes segmentation or fragmentation of the nucleus (5–7 per cent) and also vacuolization of nuclei of the lymphocytes and monocytes. There was amitosis in the monocytes. The total number of disintegrating cells (cytolysis) increased to 10 per cent as against the normal value of 1–3 per cent.

In the dogs which withstood the acute period of intoxication there was a gradual return to normal of the white blood picture. The number of lymphocytes increased with the appearance of eosinophils and a slow fall in monocytes.

The disturbances in the processes of erythropoiesis in acute poisoning were apparently deeper although in the acute period manifest only in temporary reduction in the number of polychromatophilic erythrocytes and reticulocytes. One to two months after acute poisoning both surviving dogs showed a fall in the number of erythrocytes and haemoglobin. In dog. No. 9, in which a very severe picture of intoxication was observed, the anaemia was progressive and the number of erythrocytes two months after poisoning fell to 3,440,000 per mm^3 and the haemoglobin fell to 50 per cent. The number of reticulocytes was comparatively low.

Thus, with acute single poisoning with U_3O_8 we observed depression of the processes of leucopoiesis and also symptoms of disturbance in neutrophilic leucopoiesis (shift to the right with leucocytosis). As shown by subsequent observations the changes in the white blood in the dogs were of a reversible character.

The depression of erythropoiesis was manifest in the acute period in a fall in the number of reticulocytes and, subsequently, led to more or less severe anaemia.

In conclusion, it should be noted that in evaluating the haematological findings it is necessary to take into consideration the complex character of the effect of uranium on the body. Although the direct cause of death of the animals on administration of large amounts of U_3O_8 as shown by the histological investigations of Tolgskaya (this volume, pp. 120–135) was renal insufficiency, in the majority of the animals we found, in addition, damage to the lungs in the form of necrotic panbronchitis with signs of perifocal catarrhal pneumonia. The fact that the pneumonia was due to the action of the product administered was shown by controls in which intratracheal administration of saline did not produce any pathological changes. The onset of catarrhal pneumonia is characteristic of poisoning with uranium, as noted by many workers including Novikova (1959) who observed it even for subcutaneous injection of soluble uranium salts. It is possible that the neutrophilic leucocytosis appearing on administration of large amounts of U_3O_8 into the trachea is due to an inflammatory process in the lungs.

In addition, it is also necessary to bear in mind that although uranium does not have a high specific activity it may stay in the body for a long time and the heavily ionizing alpha radiation may influence the haemopoietic system. Thus, for example, it is possible that radiation may be responsible for the destruction of the lymphoid elements found by Tolgskaya close to the conglomerations of U_3O_8 particles in the lymph nodes. It is also known that involvement of the kidneys is often accompanied by progressive anaemia of the hyporegenerative type (Tareyev, 1929; Vlados, 1950; Kassirskii and Alekseyev, 1959).

Summary

1. After oral administration of U_3O_8 (100 mg/kg 5–6 times a week for 2–4 months) the condition of the dogs remained good. The blood changes were insignificant and essentially expressed in some increase in the absolute number of lymphocytes and monocytes.

2. Repeat intratracheal administration of U_3O_8 in doses not causing symptoms of intoxication (to a total of 10–20 mg per kg animal weight) produced more or less marked absolute lymphopenia and periodic monocytosis and eosinophilia. In the majority of the animals we observed moderate neutrophilic leucocytosis. Disturbance in leucopoiesis was indicated by the cytological changes in the leucocytes; an increase in the fragmentation of the neutrophils and vacuolization of the nuclei of the lymphocytes and monocytes.

3. With acute single poisoning of the dogs with U_3O_8 via the trachea they developed leucocytosis but the shift to the right and the increase in fragmentation of the nucleus of the neutrophils suggests disturbance in leucopoiesis. This was accompanied by sharp absolute and relative lymphopenia, eosinopenia and monocytosis. Considerable cytological changes were observed (segmentation of the monocytes, vacuolization of the nuclei of the lymphocytes and monocytes, amitotic forms of division of monocytes) indicating disturbances in the formation of lymphocytes and monocytes. In the acute period of intoxication there was a sharp fall in polychromasia with disappearance of the reticulocytes which indicates depressed erythropoiesis.

4. The signs of disturbance in leucopoiesis after single acute poisoning with U_3O_8 disappeared comparatively rapidly. Erythropoiesis apparently was disturbed to a considerable extent, which may subsequently lead to development of anaemia.

References

KASSIRSKII I. A. and ALEKSEYEV G. A., *Clinical Haematology (Klinicheskaya gematologiya)*. Moscow (1959).

MAYNARD E. A. and HODGE H. C., Studies of Toxicity of Various Uranium Compounds when Fed to Experimental Animals. In: *Pharmacology and Toxicology of Uranium Compounds*, Vol. I, pp. 309–376 (Editors Voegtlin C. and Hodge H. C.). McGraw-Hill, New York (1949).

NOVIKOVA A. P., Morphological Changes in the Late Period on Exposure to Certain Radioactive Products (Morfologicheskiya izmeneniya v otdalennom periode vozdeistviya nekotorykh radioaktivnykh produktov). *Late Sequelae of Injuries Caused by Ionizing Radiations (Otdalennye posledeistviya porazhenii, vyzannykh ioniziruyushchei radiatsei)*. Moscow (1959).

ORCUTT J. A., Toxicology of Compounds of Uranium following Applications to the Skin. In: *Pharmacology and Toxicology of Uranium Compounds*, Vol. I, pp. 377–414 (Editors Voegtlin C. and Hodge H. C.). McGraw-Hill, New York (1949).

STOKINGER H. E., ROTHSTEIN A., ROBERTS E., SPIEGL C. J., DYGERT H. P., LA BELLE C. W. and SPRAGUE G. F., Toxicity following Inhalation. In: *Pharmacology and Toxicology of Uranium Compounds*, Vol. I, pp. 423–524 (Editors Voegtlin C. and Hodge H. C.). McGraw-Hill, New York (1949).

TAREYEV, YE. M., *Bright's Anaemia (Anemiya braitikov)*. Moscow (1929).

VLADOS KH. D., Practical Application of Anaemia Classifications (Prakticheskoye primeneniye klassifikatsii anemii). *Sovet. med.* **9**, 14–17 (1950).

THE EFFECT OF U_3O_8 ON THE BODY OF THE PREGNANT FEMALE AND THE FOETUS

E. B. KURLYANDSKAYA

THE effect of virtually insoluble uranous-uranic oxide (U_3O_8) on the body of the pregnant animal and foetal development is of considerable interest. The investigations of Rubanovskaya (this volume, pp. 87–100) have shown that when the poorly soluble compound containing as much as 85 per cent of the pure metal is introduced into the animal body via different routes, after a short time interval uranium begins to circulate in the blood, accumulating in low amounts in the organs and is eliminated via the excretory passages. These findings indicate that, on the one hand, conditions are present in the body for the conversion of a certain amount of U_3O_8 into a soluble state and, on the other, transfer of small particles by phagocytes through the lymphatic and circulatory systems is probable. These findings suggest that uranium may penetrate in certain amounts through the placental barrier into the foetus.

The passage of metals (iron, copper, mercury, lead, calcium, strontium, caesium, ruthenium, etc.) through the placenta is known from the literature. Thus, in the Institute of Labour Hygiene and Occupational Diseases of the U.S.S.R. Academy of Medical Sciences, Zolotareva established that mercury administered to animals and also entering the body of women factory workers is found in the tissues of the placenta and foetus and in the urine and blood of the mother.

In particular, many investigations have been devoted to penetration into the body of the foetus in the pre-natal and in the post-natal period of radioactive strontium and calcium (Pecher and Pecher, 1941; Finkel, 1947; Tutt and Vaughan, 1949; Kidman, Tutt and Vaughan, 1950; Rubanovskaya and Ushakova, 1957; Kurlyandskaya, Beloborodova and Baranova, 1957; Balabukha and Fradkin, 1958; Novikova and Burykina, 1961; Parfenov, 1960; Levchenko and Parfenov, 1962; and others).

The results obtained by these workers show that Sr and Ca readily penetrate the placenta to the foetus and that Sr and Ca are transmitted to the baby in considerable amounts in the milk of the lactating female. The placenta is readily permeable to caesium (Kurlyandskaya, Beloborodova and Baronova, 1957; Kulikova, 1959) and to iron (Kulikova, 1959). Ruthenium (Kulikova, 1959) and plutonium (Wilkinson and Hoecker, 1955; Marsden, 1959; Rysina and Tseveleva, 1962) are able to travel across the placenta only to a limited degree.

Thus, the degree of passage of various elements through the placenta depends on the atomic number, the physicochemical and biological properties, the time of pregnancy of the female and the rhythm and duration of entry. Substances least able to pass across the placenta are those with a high atomic number and those forming in biological media compounds poorly penetrating biological barriers (plutonium, uranium, etc.).

We set out to study the permeability of the placenta in relation to U_3O_8, the possibility of its excretion by the mammary glands and also the effect of this compound on embryonic development in the intrauterine and early extrauterine period.

Content of Uranium in the Tissues of the Placenta and Embryos and in the Organs of the Mother

Experiments were carried out in female rabbits which at different periods of pregnancy were given once or repeatedly U_3O_8 via the trachea in a dose of 0·06–0·135 g/kg or via the oesophagus in a dose of 0·15–1·8 g/kg. Dogs were also used in the experiment and were given uranium via the trachea and mouth in a dose of 0·1 to 0·5 g/kg.

The fluorescent method (as modified by Popov) was used to investigate the uranium content of the embryos (23 embryos of 13 females) at different times of pregnancy, and the organs, placenta and milk of the mother. In all cases it was found that the tissues of the embryo contained uranium in amounts amenable to determination by the fluorescent method. These amounts varied for the embryo from 0·001 to 0·07 mg per 100 mg irrespective of the mode of administration of U_3O_8 to the female. At the same time in the placenta we found the metal in an amount of 0·03–0·025 mg per 100 mg.

Table 1 shows that in the case of intratracheal and oral administration of U_3O_8 to the mother the embryo and placenta contained the substance. It was not possible to establish a relation between the amount of uranium contained in the placenta and the tissues of the embryo and the time of pregnancy. There was no strict relation between the amount of U_3O_8 introduced and the content of uranium in the organs (Table 2).

Our investigations showed that in the presence of uranium in the tissues of the embryo the organs and milk of the mother also contained this substance. As Table 2 shows, the milk of rabbits contained 0·008 to

TABLE 1. *Content of Uranium in Tissues of Embryos, Placenta and Milk of Females*

Route of administration	Dose in g/kg	Schedule of administration of U_3O_8 before parturition	Time of pregnancy in days	Content of uranium in mg per 100 mg		
				Foetus	Placenta	Milk of female
Intra-tracheal	0·1	Once in 4 days	30	0·021	—	0·44
Ditto	0·1	Ditto	30	0·01	—	0·44
Ditto	0·1	Ditto	30	0·012	—	0·44
Ditto	0·5	Once in 2 months	30	0·00075	—	—
Ditto	0·5	Ditto	63	0·001	—	—
Ditto	0·5	Ditto	63	0·0012	—	—
Ditto	0·1	Ditto	15	0·07	—	—
Ditto	0·15	Once in 6 days	30	0·0024	—	0·03
Ditto	0·15	Ditto	30	0·0021	—	0·03
Ditto	0·15	Ditto	30	0·0025	—	0·03
Ditto	0·125	Once in 3 months	20	0·0025	0·02	—
Ditto	0·125	Ditto	20	0·003	0·02	—
Ditto	0·125	Ditto	20	0·0065	0·02	—
Ditto	1·8	Every other day for 34 days	30	0·001	—	—
Oral	0·5	Twice in 4 days	30	0·001	0·012	0·008
Ditto	0·5	Once in 3 days	17	0·027	0·016	—
Ditto	0·25	Three times in 10 days	20	0·006	0·003	—
Ditto	0·5	Once in 2 days	30	0·014	—	0·06
Ditto	0·5	Ditto	30	0·015	—	0·06
Ditto	0·25	15 times in 34 days	30	0·007	—	—
Ditto	0·25	Ditto	30	0·0015	0·0015	—

TABLE 2. *Content of Uranium (in mg %) in Organs and Excreta of Female and Embryonic Tissues on Poisoning by Mouth*

Dose of U_3O_8 in mg/kg	Times of administration before autopsy in days	Times of pregnancy	Blood	Kidneys	Liver	Muscles	Spleen	Lymph nodes	Urine	Milk	Placenta	Embryo
60	10	20	—	0·2	0·3	—	—	—	—	0·008	0·012	0·0
60	6	24	0·03	0·1	0·07	0·002	0·06	0·12	0·01	—	0·016	0·027
80	2	25	—	0·3	0·1	—	—	0·14	—	0·008	0·14	0·09
80	2	25	—	0·3	0·1	—	—	0·14	—	0·008	0·08	0·08
150	10	20	0·002	0·15	0·005	—	0·083	—	0·037	—	0·003	0·006
170	2	30	0·01	0·1	0·01	—	0·18	0·06	0·05	0·06	—	0·014
200	6	30	—	0·01	0·002	—	—	—	—	—	0·0015	0·0015

0·06 mg of uranium per 100 mg. Thus, after administering U_3O_8 to pregnant females it is partially retained by the placenta, partially passes to the foetus and is also excreted in the milk.

Distribution of Uranium in the Organs of Newborn Animals

The distribution of uranium in the organs was studied in animals which had just been littered and were still not on maternal milk (rabbits and puppies). We studied the organs of 19 newborn rabbits of 4 mothers (Table 3). In each experiment we took organs from 2 animals. In addition, the analysis for the content of uranium was made on the organs of 17 puppies littered by 6 bitches. Five bitches were given U_3O_8 repeatedly intratracheally to a total of 0·1–0·5 g/kg weight. One bitch during 17 days before littering was given U_3O_8 via the gastro-intestinal tract (daily). She received in all 42·5 g (Table 4).

Tables 3 and 4 show that uranium is incorporated into the organs of the foetus. Most of it was found in the newborn rabbits in the gastric juice which usually fills the stomach of the foetus and also in the gastro-intestinal tract. As judged by the content of uranium the organs and fluids of the body of newborn puppies may be arranged in the following order: (1) gastric juice (uranium found in 100 per cent cases); (2) stomach and duodenum (88 per cent); (3) large intestine (78 per cent); (4) small intestines (78 per cent); (5) kidneys (70 per cent); (6) muscles and liver (66·6 per cent); (7) lungs (58·3 per cent); and (8) brain (30 per cent).

With our method of investigation uranium was never found in the bones. It is of interest to note that during intrauterine life the main excretory role is played not by the kidneys but by the gastro-intestinal tract as we have already observed in a study of trinitrotoluene.

In both series of experiments passage of the substance across the placenta to the foetus was established.

Distribution of Uranium in the Organs of Puppies Feeding on the Milk of Burdened Mothers

We studied the distribution of uranium in the organs of puppies feeding for different times (from 11 to 20 days after birth) on the milk of mothers burdened orally or intratracheally with U_3O_8 during the lactation period. In all we had under observation 11 puppies and 4 rabbits. In all the puppies fed on milk there was a low concentration of the substance in the organs and uranium was excreted in the urine. The organ distribution of uranium in these puppies was somewhat different from that in the embryos. Taking the number of cases in which uranium was found in the tissues of the organs and in the fluids of the body and also taking into account the content of the substance we may arrange the biological specimens in the following order: (1) urine (uranium found in 100 per cent); (2) kidneys (85 per cent); (3) small intestines (83.2 per cent); (4) stomach and lungs (80 per cent); (5) brain (67 per cent); (6) muscle (50 per cent); (7) heart (42·8 per cent); (8) large intestine (40 per cent); (9) spleen (28·2 per cent); (10) liver (14·2 per cent). Uranium was never found in the bones (with our method of uranium determination).

TABLE 3. *Content of Uranium (in mg %) in Organs and Fluids of Newborn Rabbits*

Organ or tissue	Rabbits			
	No. 8	No. 9	No. 15	No. 24
	For 8 days before littering daily received 70 mg/kg U_3O_8 orally	For 6 days before littering daily received 80 mg/kg U_3O_8 orally	For 30 days before littering received 80 mg/kg U_3O_8 six times orally	2 months before littering received a single intratracheal dose of 80 mg/kg U_3O_8
Blood	0·001	0·008	None	—
Gastric juice	0·33	0·008	"	0·01
Liver	0·01	0·02	"	None
Kidneys	0·3	0·3	0·01	—
Small intestines	0·05	0·007	None	0·03
Brain	—	—	"	0·015
Stomach and duodenum	—	—	0·015	—

Thus, in the animals feeding on the milk of the mother burdened with U_3O_8 during the lactation period it was found that the uranium was excreted in the urine and a low concentration was found in the organs. Uranium was also found in the urine and organs one month after feeding on mother's milk. In puppy No. 8 uranium was excreted in the urine and was also found in the tissues of the liver and spleen 90 days after birth (Table 4).

Uranium is excreted in the maternal milk and is transmitted through the milk to the progeny.

TABLE 4. *The Content of Uranium (in mg %) in Organs and Fluids of Newborn Puppies*[a]

Organ or tissue	Puppies of bitch No. 1 receiving by mouth 0·1g/kg U_3O_8 for 17 days at a time before littering (total administered 42·5 g)						Puppies of bitch No. 2 receiving U_3O_8 intratracheally 5 times for 2 months before birth (total 0·5 g/kg)		Puppies of bitches receiving U_3O_8: Single intratracheal dose of 0·1 g/kg 6 days before littering (bitch No. 3)		Puppies of bitches receiving U_3O_8: Two intratracheal doses of 100 mg 17 days before littering (bitch No. 4)	Puppies of bitch No. 7 receiving 0·1 g/kg U_3O_8 intratracheally 5 times for 14 months before littering			
	No. 1	No. 2	No. 3	No. 5	No. 6	No. 7	No. 8	No. 9	No. 10	No. 11	No. 12	No. 13	No. 14	No. 15	No. 16
Blood	None	None	—	None	None	—	—	—	—	—	None	0·0027	0·0027	—	—
Gastric juice	—	—	—	—	—	—	—	—	—	—	0·035	—	—	—	—
Liver	0·003	0·0025	None	None	0·008	None	0·005	0·02	0·002	0·001	0·005	0·0017	0·003	None	—
Kidneys	None	0·006	None	None	0·014	0·007	0·04	0·04	0·012	0·012	0·005	0·0016	0·0016	0·0016	0·0016
Small intestines	0·015	0·035	0·005	0·05	0·01	0·002	0·0035	—	0·005	0·03	None	0·012	0·0034	0·001	None
Brain	None	None	None	None	None	None	0·018	0·04	0·001	0·001	None	0·004	—	—	0·0016
Muscles	0·014	0·015	None	0·02	None	0·04	0·004	0·02	0·02	0·02	None	—	—	—	—
Heart	0·0034	—	None	0·004	None	None	0·038	0·02	0·016	0·016	None	None	None	—	0·0025
Spleen	0·016	—	—	None	None	0·025	0·041	0·07	0·05	0·05	None	—	—	—	—
Stomach and duodenum	0·006	—	—	0·0064	—	0·053	0·021	—	—	—	—	—	—	—	—
Lungs	0·003	0·0025	None	None	0·002	None	0·0011	0·02	0·007	0·009	None	—	—	—	0·0025
Milk of female	0·0012	—	—	—	—	—	0·075	0·005	—	—	—	—	—	—	—
Large intestine	0·027	0·025	0·006	0·007	0·061	—	—	—							

[a]The table gives the findings lation in reto five bitches and 15 puppies.

Effect of Chronic Burdening on the Ability of the Female to Multiply

We kept under prolonged observation (from 7 to 20 months) 8 bitches given U_3O_8 intratracheally in a dose of 0·1–0·5 g/kg and 2 who received the substance orally. In addition, observations were made on 17 rabbits of which 14 were given orally and 3 given intratracheally 0·1 to 0·15 g of uranous-uranic oxide per kg of weight. Six bitches were first exposed in the period of pregnancy 6–20 days before birth. All gave birth to quite well-formed puppies. In subsequent observations for 20 months in conditions of continued administration only 2 of the 6 bitches littered again. Of the 4 which for a long period carried U_3O_8 in the lungs, 2 became pregnant for the first time one year after the start of administration but pregnancy was interrupted spontaneously. Two others littered on one occasion. The control bitches in the period of observation littered twice. Thus, in dogs under conditions of chronic exposure to uranous-uranic oxide there was a certain tendency for parturition to decline. All the rabbits chronically administered U_3O_8 and observed for 6 months each littered on two occasions. Consequently, in the rabbits during 6 months parturition was not affected.

TABLE 5. *The Effect of Poisoning Dogs with* U_3O_8 *on the Survival Rate of Newborn Puppies*

Bitch No.	Period of poisoning before littering in days and route of administration of U_3O_8 (5–6 times a week 100 mg/kg at a time daily)	Total dose of U_3O_8 in g/kg	Litter number: Total born	Litter number: Died	Litter number: Survived
1	19 By mouth	4	8	4	4
2	11 By mouth	1·5	1	–	1
3	150 Intratracheally	0·5	2	2	–
4	6 Intratracheally	0·1	6	–	6
5	14 Intratracheally	0·25	1	–	1
6	20 Intratracheally	0·3	6	–	6
6	229 Intratracheally	0·3	4	3	1
7	450 Intratracheally	0·8	8	1	7
8	35 Intratracheally	0·5	2	–	2
8	450 Intratracheally	0·5	4	2	2
	Total	–	42 (100%)	12 (28·5%)	30 (71·5%)

Effect of Chronic Intoxication with U_3O_8 on Foetal Development in the Intrauterine and Early Extrauterine Periods

The observation was made on the development of the foetus in the intrauterine and early extrauterine period in dogs and rabbits subjected to chronic treatment with U_3O_8 in the amounts indicated above.

It was established that of 42 puppies born to 8 bitches, 12 died during 1–10 days after birth (i.e. 28·5 per cent), while 30 (i.e. 71·5 per cent) remained alive as shown in Table 5.

In the rabbits chronically exposed to U_3O_8 (via the mouth and intratracheally) this compound also had some effect on development of the embryo in the intrauterine and early extrauterine period (Table 6).

TABLE 6. *The Effect of Poisoning Rabbits with* U_3O_8 *on Survival Rate of Newborn Rabbits*

Rabbit No.	Dose of U_3O_8 in g/kg and route	Period of poisoning before littering in days	Number of foetuses	Of them		
				Ceased intra-uterine devel-opment	Died	Survived
1	0·4 Orally	10	9	—	—	9
2	0·4 Orally	4	3	—	—	3
3	0·4 Orally	20	5	5	—	—
4	0·4 Orally	20	5	5	—	—
5	0·4 Orally	11	7	6	—	1
6	0·4 Orally	2	6	—	1	5
7	0·4 Orally	55	3	—	1	2
8	0·4 Orally	60	8	—	2	6
9	0·125 Intratracheally	30	7	—	—	7
	Total	—	53	16	4	33

Consequently, of 53 foetuses only 33 were born quite viable (62·2 per cent) indicating that chronic exposure of the female to U_3O_8 has a certain effect on development of the foetus in the intrauterine and early extrauterine periods.

Effect of Poisoning of Rabbits with U_3O_8 in the Suckling Period on the Devclopment of the Newborn

Observations were made on the development of 15 newborn rabbits the mothers of which in the period of feeding (daily from 18 to 30 days) were poisoned with U_3O_8 orally. The results of the observations are presented in Table 7.

Of 15 newborn feeding on the milk of the poisoned mother in a period of 18 to 30 days, 12 died at the times indicated and only 3 lived longer.

TABLE 7. *Offspring of* U_3O_8 *Poisoned Rabbits and Their Survival Rate*

Rabbit No.	Dose of U_3O_8 in mg	Period of poisoning in days	Number of newborn rabbits	Of them	
				Died	Survived
10	3	25	2	1	1
50	5·1	30	4	2	2
51	3·6	25	2	2	—
31	6	18	7	7	—
Total			15	12	3

Effect of Poisoning with Uranyl Nitrate on the Development of the Foetus

Five pregnant rabbits were poisoned with uranyl nitrate in an amount of 0·5 mg per kg weight injected subcutaneously (3–4 times). The dose may be considered high since at this dose the animal was killed after 15–17 days in a poor condition. Of 30 embryos revealed at autopsy of the mothers most were found to have died in the intrauterine period and were in different stages of decomposition while seven were stillborn (Table 8).

As Table 8 shows, in the majority of embryos (77 per cent) development ceased in the intrauterine period. The embryos of the mother which was exposed to uranium in the middle of pregnancy were stillborn. Consequently, subacute poisoning with uranyl nitrate affects the development of the foetus in the intrauterine period. Our findings are similar to those obtained by Maynard and Hodge (1949), who found a reduction in the number of newborn from female rats exposed to chronic treatment with uranium nitrate.

TABLE 8. *Offspring of Rabbits Poisoned with Uranyl Nitrate and Their Development*

Animal No.	Dose in mg	Number of foetuses	Of them		
			Ceased to develop	Died	Survived
16	5·25	7	7	–	–
41	7	5	5	–	–
48	5·25	5	5	–	–
86	5·25	6	6	–	–
88	3·4	7	–	7	–
Total		30	23	7	–

Summary

1. Following oral or intratracheal administration to the pregnant animal of practically insoluble U_3O_8, uranium was found in the placenta and tissues of the embryo.

2. Uranium was found in the milk of lactating animals and in the tissues and urine of the puppies and young rabbits fed on the milk of the poisoned mother.

3. Chronic exposure of animals to U_3O_8 has an effect on their littering capacity and also on the intrauterine and early extrauterine development of the young rabbits and puppies.

References

BALABUKHA V. S. and FRADKIN G. YE., *Accumulation of Radioactive Elements in the Body and their Elimination (Nakopleniye radioaktivnykh elementov v organisme i ikh vyvedeniye)*. Moscow (1958).

FINKEL M. P., The Transmission of Radiostrontium and Plutonium from Mother to Offspring in Laboratory Animals. *Physiol. Zoology*, **20**, 405–421 (1947).

KIDMAN B., TUTT M. L. and VAUGHAN J. M., The Retention and Excretion of Radioactive Strontium and Yttrium in the Healthy Rabbit. *J. Path. Bact.* **62**, 2, 209 (1950).

KULIKOVA V. G., Penetration of Strontium, Caesium, Ruthenium and Iron Across the Placental and Mammary Barriers (O proniknovenii strontsiya, tseziya, ruteniya i zheleza cherez platsentarnyi i molochnyi bariery). *Meditsinskaya radiologiye*, **IV**, 5, 23–27 (1959).

KURLYANDSKAYA E. B., BELOVORODOVA N. L. and BARANOVA YE. F., Distribution and Excretion of Radioactive Strontium During its Continuous Oral Administration to Rabbits (Raspredeleniye i vyvedeniye radioaktivnogo strontsiya pri khronicheskom vvedenii ego krolikam cherez rot). In: *The Toxicology of Radioactive Substances (Materialy po toksikologii radioaktivnykh veshchestv)*, Vol. 1, pp. 16–23. Pergamon Press, Oxford (1962).

Kurlyandskaya E. B., Beloborodova N. L. and Baranova Ye. F., Distribution of Radioactive Caesium in the Organism and its Excretion (Raspredeleniye v organizme i vyvedeniye radioaktivnogo tseziya). In: *The Toxicology of Radioactive Substances*, Vol. 1, pp. 31–41. Pergamon Press, Oxford (1962).

Levchenko M. A. and Parfenov Yu. D., Transmission of ^{90}Sr to the Progeny of Rats after Single Intraperitoneal Administration. (Perekhod Sr^{90} k potomstvu u krys posle odnokratnogo vvedeniya). *Meditsinskaya radiologiya*, **VII**, 9, 74–77 (1962).

Marsden E., Radioactivity of Soils, Plant Ashes and Animal Bones. *Nature (London)*, **183**, 924–925 (1959).

Maynard E. A. and Hodge H. C., Studies of Toxicity of Various Uranium Compounds when Fed to Experimental Animals. In: *Pharmacology and Toxicology of Uranium Compounds*, Vol. I, pp. 309–376. (Editors Voegtlin C. and Hodge H. C.). McGraw-Hill, New York (1949).

Novikova A. P. and Burykina L. N., Aspects of the Development of the Progeny of Rats Exposed to Blastomogenic Concentrations of Strontium-90 (Ob osobennostyakh razvitiya potomstva krys, porazhennykh blastomogennymi kontsentratsiyami strontsiya-90). *Effect of Radiostrontium on the Animal Body (Vliyaniya radiostrontsiya na zhivotnyi organizm)*. Moscow (1961).

Parfenov Yu. D., Transmission of Strontium from Mother to Progeny (Perekhod strontsiya ot materi k potomstvu). *Medistinskaya, radiologiya* **5**, 10, 75–78 (1960).

Pecher Ch. and Pecher J., Radiocalcium and Radiostrontium Metabolism in Pregnant Mice. *Proc. Soc. Exp. Biol.* **46**, 1 (1941).

Rubanovskaya A. A. and Ushakova V. F., Accumulation of Radioactive Strontium in Young Rats Born to and Fed by Females Receiving Continuous Oral Administration of ^{89}Sr or a Mixture of ^{89}Sr and ^{91}Sr. In: *The Toxicology of Radioactive Substances*, Vol. 1, pp. 31–41. Pergamon Press, Oxford (1962).

Tutt M. and Vaughan J., Metabolism of Radioactive Strontium in the Rabbit. *Biochem. J.* **44**, 35 (1949).

Wilkinson P. N. and Hoecker F. E., Selective Placental Transmission of Radioactive Alkaline Earths and Plutonium. Report AECU-2400 (Kansas University).

PATHOMORPHOLOGICAL CHANGES IN ANIMALS FOLLOWING ACUTE AND CHRONIC POISONING WITH U_3O_8

M. S. TOLGSKAYA

AS FAR back as 1889, Woroschilsky described in detail the histological lesions produced by poisoning with uranium salts. From his experimental investigations on cats, dogs, rabbits and other animals given uranium nitrate and other uranium salts subcutaneously and by mouth, he concluded that uranium is very toxic. From the findings of Woroschilsky it follows that administration by any of these routes will produce sharp haemorrhagic gastroenterocolitis, parenchymatous hepatitis and pulmonary haemorrhages and oedema.

Later investigations into the toxicology of various uranium salts added little to this picture. All authors emphasize that the severest lesions occur in the kidneys (Bencosme *et al.*, 1960), being less severe in the liver. In some cases brief mention is made of lesions of the brain capillaries and tissues.

Novikova, studying the late sequelae (after 4–5 months) of acute poisoning with soluble uranium salts, concluded that small amounts of uranium appear to be retained in the body and produce prolonged processes of dystrophy and regeneration in all organs. The low specific activity is compensated by the length of exposure. Regenerative phenomena predominate in all organs and only in the spleen do dystrophic changes prevail.

In the literature there is an almost complete dearth of reports of pathomorphological findings on exposure of the internal organs to insoluble uranium salts (uranous-uranic oxide). The only report found is that of Barnett and Metcalfe whose results were published in 1949 and translated into Russian in 1951. These authors studied the changes in the internal organs of animals exposed to U_3O_8 dust. The details presented by the authors are very scanty. Pulmonary haemorrhages and oedema are described. In the kidneys a dystrophic process was found in the epithelium of the convoluted tubules in which regenerative changes appeared within only 1–2 days. In the opinion of these authors, the glomeruli are involved only in severe cases.

The purpose of the present investigation was to study the pathohistological changes in the internal organs on exposure to practically insoluble uranous-uranic oxide. The study was made on 60 animals (27 dogs and 33 rabbits) which had been subjected to acute and chronic poisoning with U_3O_8. The compound in a saline suspension was introduced by three routes into the animals: intratracheally, subcutaneously or by mouth. The life span of the animals varied from 4 to 425 days. Some animals died with signs of damage to the kidneys and uraemic coma or pneumonia, but most were in a good condition when killed by electric current (dogs) or by air embolism (rabbits). Histological studies were made of the lungs, kidneys, spleen, lymph nodes, skin and intestines. The sections were stained with haematoxylin-eosin, for fat (with Sudan), for connective tissue (by van Giesson), for iron and calcium.

The investigations may be broken down into two major groups: (1) acute poisoning with uranium by the intratracheal route; and (2) chronic poisoning with uranium by different routes.

Acute Poisoning with Uranium by the Intratracheal Route

The investigations were carried out on 10 dogs given on one occasion a large dose of uranium by a special technique of intratracheal administration using hexenal anaesthesia. With this method of administration a considerable part of the uranium enters the lung tissue (30–100 mg per kg animal weight). The life span after administration varied from 4 to 20 days.

Autopsy of the animals which died from acute intoxication revealed the following information. The mucosa of the upper respiratory tract was slightly plethoric; the lung tissue was engorged and slightly oedematous containing in places small foci of catarrhal pneumonia. Spread over all the tissue of the lungs were a fairly large number of black spots, dots and bands usually of perivascular and peribronchial localization. The broncho-pulmonary and broncho-tracheal lymph nodes on sectioning were black and solid. The mucosa of the intestines and stomach was unevenly plethoric, with here and there small petechial and larger haemorrhages. The liver was filled with blood, with damaged capsule, on sectioning the tissue was dull and greyish brown. The kidneys were slightly enlarged, the capsule easily came away, the cortical layer was swollen and greyish. The medullary substance was plethoric and oedematous with in places petechial haemorrhages.

We now describe the histological findings.

Lungs. Engorgement and minor oedema of the lung tissue. Diffuse thickening of the interalveolar septa without clear multiplication of the fibroblastic elements. The septa were thickened as a result of multiplication of large bright cells with a diffuse nucleus and basophilic protoplasm. The black uranium particles lay in piles in the peribronchial and perivascular tissue or diffusely over all the interstitial tissue of the lungs. Nodule-like conglomerations of uranium particles in the peribronchial lymph follicles were found in only one case.

Severe involvement of the bronchial tree was conspicuous. In the lumen of the small and medium bronchi we found a large number of black uranium particles lying among the leucocytes and mucus. The wall of such bronchi was considerably altered: the mucosa and submucosa were fused, and sometimes completely destroyed, so that in places all that was left of the wall were fragments of muscle fibres. Sometimes fragments of the destroyed wall and all the contents of the lumen of the bronchus escaped and the specimen showed cavities of irregular shape surrounded like "muffs" by a large number of black uranium particles (Fig. 1). In the surrounding lung tissue there were phenomena of highly marked peribronchial perifocal pneumonia often with karyorrhexis and subsequent fusion of the nuclei of the cells of the exudate. In some small vessels the wall was homogenized with small leucocytic thrombi present.

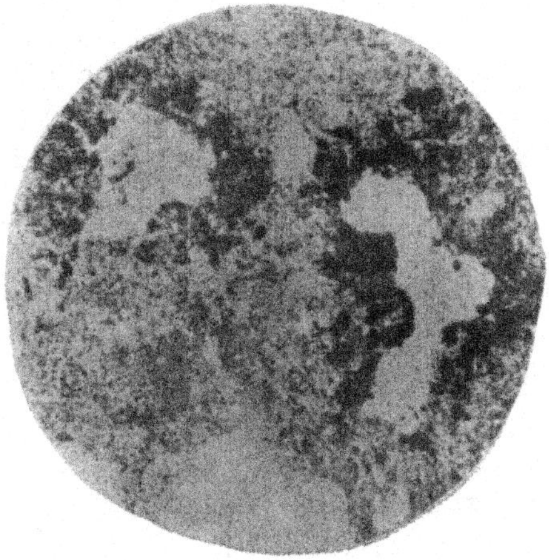

FIG. 1. Cavities at the site of the destroyed bronchi. Black particles of uranous-uranic oxide surround like "muffs" the bronchi with perifocal catarrhal pneumonia nearby (dog, 5 days after single administration)

In places there was very pronounced oedema of the perivascular tissue around the small and medium vessels. In one case (an animal living longer after poisoning) solitary foci of hyperplasia of the mucosa of the large bronchi were seen with metaplasia of the epithelium of the bronchi at these sites, where it was high, multi-layered and with a picture reminiscent of polyposis.

Lymph nodes and spleen. In the broncho-pulmonary and tracheo-bronchial lymph nodes there was considerable depletion of lymphoid elements, and karyorrhexis of the nuclei of the lymphocytes. A picture of marked catarrhal-desquamative sinusitis was observed with multiplication of bright reticulo-endothelial cells. Black U_3O_8 grains lay freely in the sinuses and under the capsule of the nodes (Fig. 2) or within the large bright cells in which karyorrhexis of the nuclei was also often visible. In the spleen and other lymph nodes the lymphoid elements were sparse particularly within the follicles with multiplication of large bright cells of the sinuses with symptoms of catarrhal-desquamative sinusitis, clearly marked erythrophagia, formation of large cells of the megakaryocyte type and severe haemosiderosis of the organ.

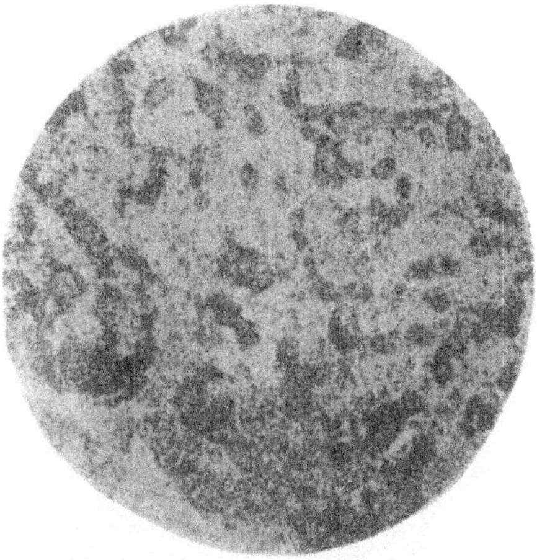

FIG. 2. Broncho-pulmonary lymph node. Reduction in the number of lymphoid elements. Catarrhal-desquamative sinusitis. Black particles of uranous-uranic oxide lie beneath the capsule of the lymph node (dog, 12 days after single administration)

Kidneys. A large number of hyaline cylinders in the lumens of the convoluted tubules (Fig. 3). Marked dystrophy of the epithelium of the tubules in the form of protein swelling and fine-droplet fatty degeneration of the protoplasm. In places necroses of solitary convoluted tubules. At the site of the dead convoluted tubules all that was visible were homogeneous, structureless, pink protein masses with partial or complete encrustation by calcium salts (Fig. 4). The stroma of the kidney proliferated around such dead masses. The lumens of the capsules of some glomeruli were considerably distended and filled with serous (sometimes containing protein) or haemorrhagic fluid. The glomeruli had an increased number of nuclei, here and there compressed as it were by fluid present in the lumen

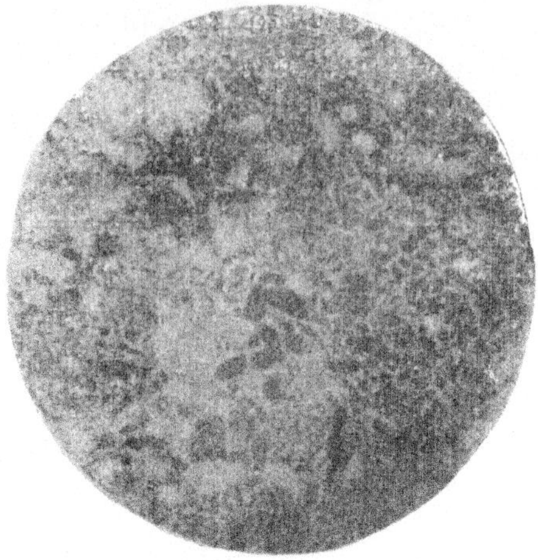

FIG. 3. Large number of hyaline cylinders in the lumen of the renal convoluted tubules (dog, 7 days after single administration)

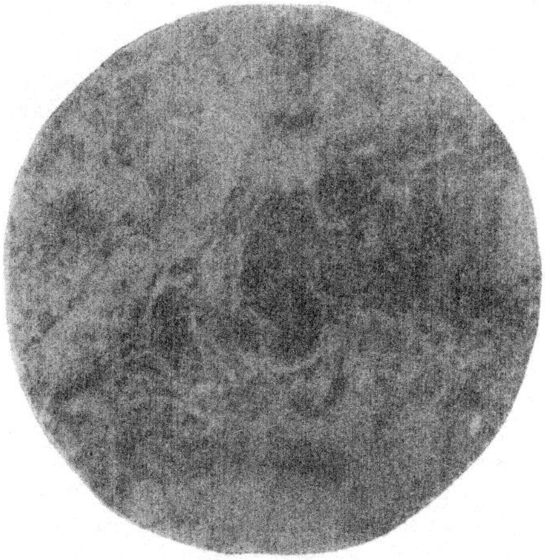

FIG. 4. Structureless protein mass at the site of dead convoluted tubules (dog, 10 days after single administration). Partial encrustation of it by calcium salts

of the capsule. In the animals living for a shorter time after poisoning the involvement of the glomeruli was more distinctly marked.

Liver. Solitary hepatic cells with swollen and vacuolized protoplasm. Bi-, tri-, and tetra-nucleated hepatic cells were encountered (as a sign of atypical regeneration). Multiplication of the reticulo-endothelial cells was observed sometimes with fine-droplet fatty dystrophy of their protoplasm and nuclear pycnosis. Heavier damage was shown by the liver cells in animals living for a long time after intoxication.

Summing up the results of microscopic study of the organs of the group of dogs with acute intratracheal intoxication with U_3O_8, we may conclude that intratracheal administration of a high dose of U_3O_8 produces in the lungs severe changes with considerable impairment of the bronchi in the form of desquamative or necrotic bronchitis with signs of peribronchial, perifocal and microfocal pneumonia, with solitary leucocytic thrombi in the small vessels, sometimes with homogenization of the walls of the small vessels and with accumulation of U_3O_8 grains in the perivascular and peribronchial tissue in the form of a "muff". No nodule-like conglomerations of U_3O_8 were found in the lungs of dogs in most cases. We noted diffuse thickening of the interalveolar septa through swelling of the tissue, minor infiltration by leucocytes and multiplying large bright cells without clear multiplication of fibroblastic elements.

No less severe changes were found in all animals in the kidney tissue expressed in marked focal necrotic nephrosis and extracapillary serous and serofibrinous glomerulitis. These observations were confirmed by the clinical findings as most of the animals died with signs of renal insufficiency.

In the regional broncho-pulmonary lymph nodes we saw U_3O_8 grains and heavy depletion of the lymphoid elements with proliferation of the reticulo-endothelial cells with signs of catarrhal-desquamative sinusitis. A similar reduction in the lymphoid elements and less marked multiplication of the reticulo-endothelial cells were found in the peripheral lymph nodes and spleen.

In the liver, in all cases, we observed a moderate dystrophic process with swelling and vacuolization of the protoplasm of the hepatic cells. In some cases we observed fine-droplet fatty dystrophy of the protoplasm of the hepatic cells and multiplication of the reticulo-endothelial cells often followed by pycnosis of their nuclei and fatty dystrophy of their protoplasm. In addition, in the hepatic cells we noticed moderate regeneration with formation of misshapen multinucleate forms.

Chronic Poisoning with U_3O_8 by Different Routes of Administration

The total number of animals used was 34 (15 dogs and 19 rabbits), the life span was from 30 to 425 days. All the animals were in a good general condition when killed. This group may be divided into three subgroups:

(A) Intratracheal administration of uranium in 11 rabbits and 7 dogs.
(B) Subcutaneous injection of uranium in 6 rabbits.
(C) Oral administration of uranium to 8 dogs and 2 rabbits.

Intratracheal Administration

Eleven rabbits received via the lungs a small single injection of uranium (from 30 to 100 mg per kg weight) after which the animals were in a good state from 250 to 315 days.*

For 30–60 days 7 dogs received repeatedly high intratracheal doses of uranium (from 300 to 500 mg/kg). However, the uranium was not given under hexenal anaesthesia and much of it was lost by coughing. The investigations of Rubanovskaya (this volume, p.93) showed that only 5–8 per cent of the U_3O_8 given, reached the lungs. On administration of the compound the animals remained in a good condition for a long time and were killed after 70–425 days.

At autopsy of the animals of the whole subgroup there were no deviations from normal visible to the naked eye in the parenchymatous organs. In the lung tissue of the rabbits scattered foci of small black nodules about the size of a pinhead or smaller were seen, often around the vessels and bronchi.

Microscopic examination of the internal organs of the rabbits gave the following results.

Lungs. In places considerable thickening of the interalveolar septa were observed which contained many large bright cells and a few fibroblastic elements. Black U_3O_8 grains were concentrated in the perivascular and peribronchial tissue of the lungs. Over the pulmonary tissue, usually around the vessels and bronchi, were a large number of black nodule-like formations, regular and round, consisting in the main of black particles, a small number of lymphoid elements and a considerable number of large bright cells with basophilic protoplasm and a diffuse nucleus. These nodule-like formations were separated by a thin connective tissue capsule from the surrounding lung tissue but no considerable growth of tissue was seen around and within the nodule-like formations (Fig. 5). Bright large cells with basophilic protoplasm and diffuse nucleus surrounded the black clumps of uranium and sometimes contained in the protoplasm black uranium granules. Often necrobiotic changes were also observed in these large cells in the form of karyorrhexis of their nuclei and dissolution of the protoplasm with formation of cell ghosts. In some nodule-like formations among the black uranium grains were blue grains of calcium deposited at the site of the dead cells.

Nodule-like formations were encountered in which all the cellular ele-

*The animals of this group were arbitrarily assigned to the group of chronically burdened since for 250–315 days they bore practically insoluble U_3O_8.

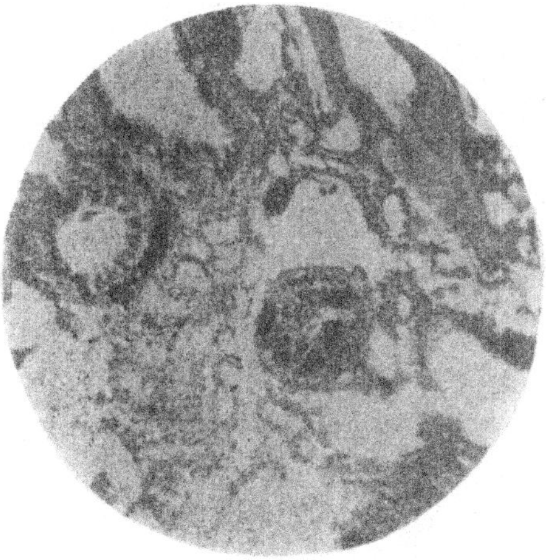

FIG. 5. Conglomeration of uranium in peribronchial tissue. Nodule of bright cells and black grains of uranous-uranic oxide (rabbit, 255 days after single administration)

ments were destroyed and the uranium grains filled the whole nodule. In some nodules as well as large bright cells and uranium grains we observed large giant cells with a large number of nuclei and in the surrounding lung tissue highly marked desquamation of the alveolar epithelium without sharp fibrosis of the tissue. In one case we observed mild focal hyperplasia and metaplasia of the mucosal epithelium of a large bronchus. The epithelium of the bronchus was in places tall and cubic and was arranged in 2–3 layers suggestive of polypous proliferation.

In some cases (with a life span of up to 315 days) the lymphoid elements almost completely disappeared from the bronchial lymph nodes with considerable growth of the connective tissue along with multiplication of the bright, large reticulo-endothelial cells. In the peripheral lymph nodes and spleen there was heavy impoverishment of lymphoid elements associated with signs of catarrhal-desquamative sinusitis with multiplication of reticulo-endothelial elements, sometimes with pycnosis of their nuclei and sclerosis and haemosiderosis of the organ. In addition, sometimes erythrophagia and the appearance of large cells of the megacaryocyte type were observed.

Kidneys. Swelling of the epithelium of the individual convoluted tubules was seen with fine-droplet fatty dystrophy of the epithelium of solitary ones. The greatest changes in the tubules were found between the cortical and medullary layers. Sometimes focal regeneration of the tubular epithelium was seen in the form of cells with mitotic figures.

Liver. The lesions were slight. Occasionally we noted uneven staining of the protoplasm of the hepatic cells, swelling and vacuolization and the appearance of bi- and trinucleated hepatic cells as signs of abnormal regeneration. The juvenile hepatic cells in places disturbed the regular form of the liver cords. There was very heavy multiplication of the reticulo-endothelial cells, sometimes with pycnosis of their nuclei and fine droplet fatty degeneration of the protoplasm (Fig. 6).

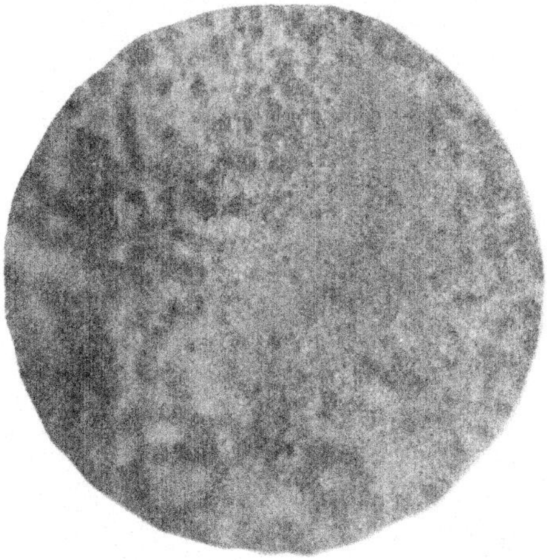

FIG. 6. Hyperplasia of the reticulo-endothelial elements in the liver. Swelling of the protoplasm of hepatic cells (rabbit, 315 days after single administration)

Microscopic examination of the internal organs of the dogs revealed changes differing from those noted above in rabbits only in that they were less intense. However, it should be noted that microscopic inspection of the lungs of the dogs did not indicate any nodule-like conglomerations of black particles. All we noted was plethora of the lung tissue and thickening of the interalveolar septa without sharp development of fibrosis and also a low content of black U_3O_8 particles in the thickened septa. The reason would appear to be that on intratracheal injection of uranium more of it was removed by coughing in dogs than in rabbits. No nodule-like conglomerations of U_3O_8 particles were seen in the lymph follicles of the lung tissue in dogs in which we observed a slight microfocal dystrophic process in the epithelium of the renal tubules and liver cells with weakly marked regeneration. Apparently the low doses of uranium on being absorbed in the lungs maintained the dystrophic process in the liver and kidneys, which proceeded for a long time without any tendency to abate and was accompanied by the same weakly marked prolonged regeneration.

SUBCUTANEOUS INJECTION

This group comprised 6 rabbits, 4 of which were injected subcutaneously with 1·4 g U_3O_8. On the 210th day the animals were killed in a good condition. The other rabbits were injected subcutaneously with large doses of U_3O_8 (2·5–3·2 g). After 60 and 180 days the animals were killed in a severe condition. At autopsy of this subgroup no gross lesions were detected in the internal organs of the majority of animals. The lung tissue was free of any foci of compaction and filled normally with blood. The gastro-intestinal mucosa was also filled normally with blood. The spleen, the kidney and the liver were macroscopically free of pathological lesions. The skin at the site of administration of uranium was not ulcerated and the hair cover was intact. In the subcutaneous tissue there were large black masses of U_3O_8 with no oedema or infiltrates in the vicinity. From the black masses ran thin black bands towards the regional lymph nodes which were solid and on sectioning black. In the two cases with subcutaneous injection of large doses the liver and kidneys were macroscopically dullish and in places greyish.

In this group the greatest changes were observed at the site of administration in the subcutaneous fatty tissue where among the connective tissue in the lymph fissures freely lay grains and clumps of U_3O_8. There was well-marked clumpy disintegration of the fibres of the adjacent muscles. Thrombosis of the small veins was rarely noticed and even less often swelling of the walls of the small vessels. No distinct infiltrative reaction around the substance introduced was noted; there were only small foci of multiplication of histiocytic elements (Fig. 7). The skin above the site of injection was unchanged. Heavy damage was sustained by the regional lymph nodes where a large amount of the product accumulated, leading to destruction of the lymphoid and multiplication of reticulo-endothelial elements of the node. Where there was a high content of U_3O_8 in the regional lymph nodes the tissue was almost entirely replaced by black masses. In the other lymph nodes and spleen there was a distinct dystrophic process in the form of karyorrhexis of the nuclei of the lymphoid elements with destruction of cells and reduction in the lymphoid tissue even within the follicles and multiplication of reticulo-endothelial cells.

In the majority of cases we observed a very weakly marked microfocal dystrophic process of the epithelium of the renal tubules and hepatic cells and also a weakly marked process of regeneration. In the liver, in addition, multiplication of reticulo-endothelial cells was seen, sometimes with pycnosis of their nuclei.

The dystrophic process in the liver and kidneys went on for a long time without any tendency to abate. The process of regeneration also proceeded quietly but stubbornly and the animal was virtually healthy. In the 2 rabbits

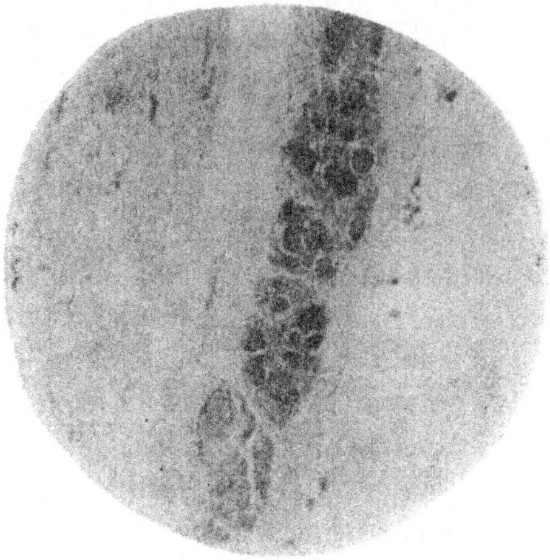

FIG. 7. Clumpy disintegration of muscle fibres with sclerosis and histiocytic infiltrates around (rabbit, 180 days after administration)

given the large doses of U_3O_8 the dystrophic changes in the liver and kidneys were more sharply marked.

In all cases practically no changes were seen in the lungs except for minor swelling and thickening of the alveolar septa. As compared with the group of animals with intratracheal administration the dystrophic changes in the internal organs on subcutaneous injection of U_3O_8 were less sharply marked. The reason would appear to be that less uranium was absorbed from the black particles lying under the skin than from those in the lung tissue by the intratracheal route. Only where the animals bore under the skin very high doses of U_3O_8 were the dystrophic changes in the liver and kidneys more intense.

ORAL ADMINISTRATION OF URANIUM

This group contained 10 animals (8 dogs and 2 rabbits daily given U_3O_8 by mouth, 100 mg per kg weight). Burdening lasted for 30–50 days. The total amount of U_3O_8 fed to the animals was on average 16–33 g. Only one dog received 100 g of the compound in 50 days. All the animals were killed in good condition. At autopsy no sharp gross deviations from normal were noted in the internal organs in this group. In the lungs there was minor plethora. The mucosa of the gastro-intestinal tract was unevenly plethoric; in the liver, kidneys and spleen no deviations from normal were noted macroscopically. Histological inspection revealed only uneven plethora in the gastro-intestinal mucosa and submucosa in all animals. Only for large doses of U_3O_8 were isolated small haemorrhages observed in the mucosa and submucosa and sometimes thrombi in the small veins. The changes in the liver and kidneys in all cases except those receiving large doses were negligible. The dystrophic process was weaker than for other routes of administration since apparently the bulk of the product is passed out of the body without being absorbed in the gut. High doses gave a negligible dystrophic process in liver and kidneys accompanied by the same feeble process of regeneration. The special features of the process in the liver for high

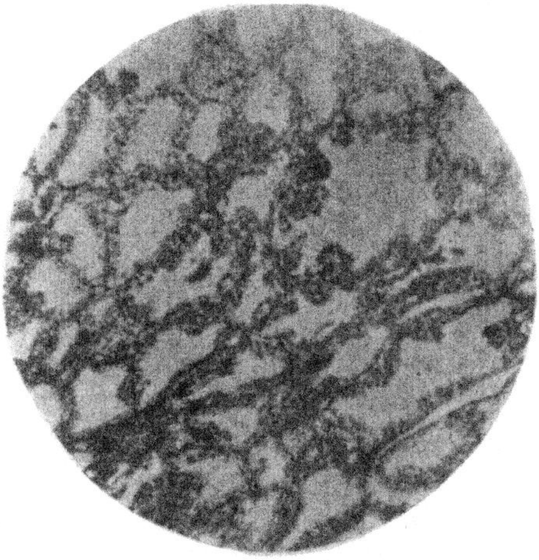

FIG. 8. Papillomatous proliferation of the epithelium of the follicles. Absence of colloid (dogs, 210 days, repeat administration)

doses of U_3O_8 were oedema of the perivascular tissue of the liver and widening of the perivascular lymph spaces and also fatty dystrophy of the endothelium of the vessels of the liver and epithelium of the bile capillaries. These symptoms were particularly marked in animals where after chronic oral intoxication high doses of the compound were also given intratracheally.

The lymph nodes and spleen displayed signs of catarrhal-desquamative sinusitis and moderate multiplication of bright large reticulo-endothelial cells without appreciable depletion of lymphoid elements.

In addition to the above investigations we studied the morphological changes in the thyroid and nervous system produced by acute and chronic U_3O_8 intoxication.

We studied the pathomorphological changes in the thyroids of 22 dogs exposed to acute and chronic intoxication with U_3O_8. In 10 dogs with intratracheal injection of uranium (killed from 30 to 210 days after injection) and with oral administration (killed from 30 to 50 days after administration ceased) the same proliferative process was found in the thyroid gland which in our view is of considerable interest. There was almost complete absence of colloid in the acini. The follicles instead of being of regular round shape had irregular contours. The epithelium of the follicles displayed well-marked, papillomatous proliferations in the form of frequently branching papillae (Fig. 8). Marked cell polymorphism was observed. In some cases the epithelium of the follicles proliferated and formed strands; the vesicles were very small and often had no lumen. The general picture resembled parenchymatous goitre. The changes in the dogs injected intratracheally were more marked.

We studied the pathomorphological changes in the nervous system of 15 dogs and rabbits subjected to acute and chronic intoxication with U_3O_8. The material may be broken down into two groups.

First group. Acute intratracheal intoxication with U_3O_8 with a life span from 4 to 20 days after administration. Autopsy of the animals showed marked plethora and oedema of the cerebrum and pia mater.

Microscopic inspection revealed in the brain highly pronounced plethora with stases in the small vessels and capillaries, signs of perivascular and pericellular oedema, numerous minor haemorrhages with swollen and sometimes homogenized walls of the small vessels. Hyaline thrombi were sometimes found in the vessels. Around some vessels there were deposits of iron-containing pigment, with multiplication of the glia and microglia around the vessels and nerve cells with acute swelling of the protoplasm of the nerve cells of the various layers of the cortex. The pyramidal cells of the third layer of the cortex were sometimes round as a result of heavy swelling of the protoplasm. The cell processes were thick, and visible a long way from the cell. The nuclei in some swollen cells were shifted to the side, the tigroid matter was dissolved at the centre but preserved at some points of the cell periphery. In the protoplasm of some cells small vacuoles were well visible. Vacuolization of the protoplasm in the round cells of the second and fourth layers of the cortex was particularly well marked. In the subcortical ganglia, the thalamo-hypothalamic region and the medulla oblongata the dystrophic process in the nerve cells was much more sharply marked and consisted in total chromatolysis and sharper vacuolization of the protoplasm (Fig. 9).

Second group. Chronic single and repeat intratracheal U_3O_8 injection in dogs with a life span from 70 to 425 days. A notable feature at autopsy was the slight plethora and insignificant oedema of the brain and pia mater.

Microscopic examination disclosed in the brain homogenization and swelling of capillary walls. Deposition of droplets of fat in the endothelium of the capillaries, sometimes hyalinosis of the walls of the small vessels, solitary minor haemorrhages, multiplication of glial elements around the vessels with in places perivascular oedema. The nerve cells of the various sections of the brain were altered. In the cortex, we saw swollen transillumi-

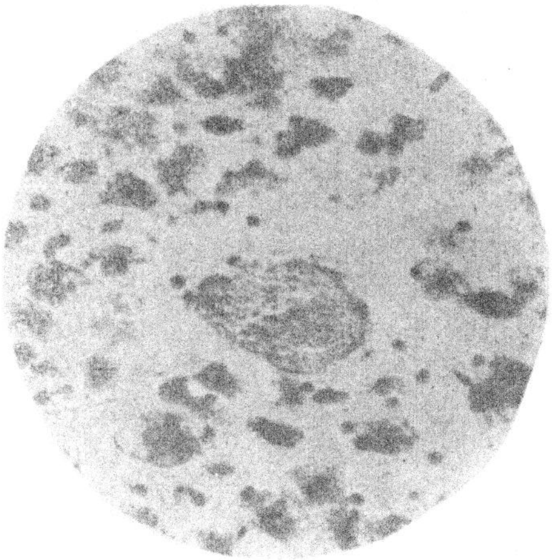

FIG. 9. Vacuolization of protoplasm of cells of thalamic region of brain (dog, 20 days, repeat administration)

nated cells with a large number of small vacuoles in the protoplasm. Here and there, in the third layer of the cortex were groups of shrivelled darkly stained cells. More marked changes were found in the subcortical ganglia of the thalamo-hypothalamic region and in the medulla oblongata. Here it was possible to find cells with heavily vacuolized protoplasm. Swollen cells came into view with dissolution of tigroid matter at the centre and maintenance of it only at the cell periphery. Sometimes phenomena of caryocytolysis were seen with formation of cell ghosts next to which were dark, shrivelled cells. In the protoplasm of some cells deposits of fat droplets were observed. There was heavy multiplication of the cells of the microglia and oligodendroglia accumulated around the changed nerve cells, often with penetration of glial elements within the body of a nerve cell, which many workers interpret as neuronophagia. In places there was focal multiplication of the microglia with multiplication of astrocytes around the vessels. The process was of distinct focal character, i.e. next to the damaged cells it was always possible to observe groups of quite normal cells.

Summary

1. On acute intratracheal intoxication with U_3O_8 for a life span from 4 to 20 days we found in the lungs desquamative and necrotic bronchitis, sometimes with destruction of the wall of the bronchus, signs of catarrhal peribronchial pneumonia, perivascular and peribronchial muff-like conglomerations of U_3O_8 grains and diffuse thickening of the interalveolar septa without formation of nodules in the lung tissue. We noted focal necrotic nephrosis, extracapillary, serofibrinous glomerulitis and moderate pro-

tein dystrophy of the hepatic cells. In the lymph nodes and spleen there was a sharp reduction in the number of lymphoid elements and multiplication of the reticulo-endothelial cells of the sinuses.

2. On chronic intratracheal U_3O_8 intoxication in an experiment lasting from 250 to 315 days we saw in the lungs deposition of U_3O_8 about the bronchi and vessels in the form of round nodule-like formations. At the centre of the nodule it was sometimes possible to observe signs of necrosis. In some cases focal hyperplasia and metaplasia of the bronchial epithelium were observed. In the lymph nodes and spleen almost complete disappearance of lymphoid elements and multiplication of reticulo-endothelial elements was established. In the kidneys there was protein dystrophy of the epithelium of the tubules and in the liver slight dystrophic changes in the cells, signs of regeneration and formation of tri- and tetranucleated liver cells and heavy multiplication of reticulo-endothelial cells.

3. On subcutaneous injection of U_3O_8 in an experiment lasting up to 210 days, in the subcutaneous fatty tissue (at the site of injection) we found free-lying black U_3O_8 grains without a clear infiltrative reaction in the vicinity and clumpy disintegration of the fibres of the underlying muscles. In the regional lymph nodes there was a large accumulation of U_3O_8 grains and sharp reduction in the number of lymphoid elements. The liver and kidneys showed a weak dystrophic process and equally weak signs of regeneration.

4. The dystrophic changes in the internal organs on subcutaneous injection of U_3O_8 were less sharply marked than for intratracheal administration, apparently due to the slighter absorption of the product from the U_3O_8 particles deposited below the skin.

5. With chronic oral intoxication with U_3O_8 in an experiment lasting from 30–50 days we found minor haemorrhages and thrombi in the vessels of the gastro-intestinal mucosa and submucosa. The changes in the liver and kidneys were negligible. Apparently, the bulk of the U_3O_8 is absorbed only in an insignificant amount in the intestines.

6. With chronic U_3O_8 intratracheal and oral intoxication in an experiment lasting from 30 to 210 days a proliferative process was detected in the thyroid in the form of papillomatous proliferation of the follicular epithelium.

7. With acute intratracheal U_3O_8 intoxication in an experiment lasting from 4 to 20 days the brain of the animals showed perivascular and pericellular oedema, minor haemorrhages and hyaline thrombi in the vessels, acute swelling and vacuolization of the protoplasm of the cells of the second and fourth cortical layers and also more sharply marked vacuolization and chromatolysis of the cells of the thalamo-hypothalamic region.

8. With chronic U_3O_8 intoxication with a life span from 70 to 425 days the brain of the animals displayed minor perivascular haemorrhages, peri-

vascular oedema, shrivelling of cortical cells and vacuolization and caryocytolysis of the cells of the thalamo-hypothalamic region. The dystrophic changes in the nerve cells were accompanied by focal multiplication of the glial and microglial elements.

References

BARNETT T. B. and METCALFE R. G., Pathological Anatomy following Uranium Poisoning. In: *Pharmacology and Toxicology of Uranium Compounds*, Vol. 2, p. 207. (Editors Voegtlin C. and Hodge H. C.). McGraw-Hill, New York (1949).

BENCOSME S. A., STONE R. S., LATIA H. and MADDEN S. C., Acute Tubular and Glomerular Lesions in Rat Kidneys after Uranium Injury. *Arch. Path.* **69**, 470–476 (1960).

NOVIKOVA A. P., Late Sequelae of Single and Repeat Poisoning with Soluble Uranium Salts (Otdalennye posledestviya odnokratnogo i povtornogo otravleniya rastvorimymi solyami urana). Summaries of Reports to the Third All-Union Congress of Morbid Anatomists in Kharkov, Kharkov (1959)

WOROSCHILSKY J., Wirkung des Urans. Diss., Dorpat (1889).

INDEX

Printed in Dunstable, United Kingdom

91221449R00085